SHIFT
your FATE

LIFE-CHANGING WISDOM FOR PROACTIVE KIDNEY PATIENTS

RISA SIMON

SHIFT YOUR FATE
Life-Changing Wisdom
For Proactive Kidney Patients

FIRST EDITION

By Risa Simon

Disclaimer: This book is not intended to replace medical advice or recommendations by healthcare providers. Instead, it is intended to help you make informed decisions about your health by partnering with your healthcare team, so you can improve your outcome. If you suspect that you have a medical concern, it is essential to seek medical attention from a competent provider immediately.

Printed in the United States of America

United States of America Copyright Office
Registration Number TX7-655-469

ISBN 978-0-578-11363-0

FIRST PRINTING: WORLD KIDNEY DAY, MARCH 8, 2012.
REVISED: July 1, 2016

THE PROACTIVE PATH
A Division of Simon Says Seminars, Inc.

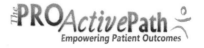

GRATITUDES

This book is dedicated to Melissa Blevins Bein, my amazing *living* kidney donor, for her selfless and heroic spirit. Melissa's *gift-of-life* allowed me to bypass dialysis so I could live my best life possible. Her passionate calling to donate a kidney to me, is what makes this remarkable experience so magical for me. I celebrate the *privilege* of being her recipient every minute of every day with immense gratitude.

I also dedicate this book to my best friend, life-partner and big-hearted husband, Wally Simon, for being my biggest fan as I was dreaming a bigger dream. His unconditional understanding of the importance of my work is what allowed me to share my message with a larger audience. I would be remiss if I didn't acknowledge his remarkable patience and bachelor skills, while I was having an affair with my computer screen and keyboard. His respect for my vision, and willingness to be my sounding board, is what allowed me to soar *beyond* the printed word.

My gratitude also goes out to my sweet brother Ryan and his loving *living* kidney donor wife, Kim, for demonstrating "in real time" the joy of living donor transplantation—for both donor and recipient. Their enthusiastic support of my transplant-first vision continues to underscore the value of getting this book into the hands of all Chronic Kidney Disease (CKD) patients.

I equally honor all the renal groups and transplant centers who are seeking improved outcomes for their patients. It is my hope that they will give all their transplant eligible patients access to this book. By doing so, they'll advance patient education and engagement, and support preemptive *(before dialysis)* transplant opportunities that can circumvent the need for dialysis.

And, of course, this book acknowledges all the CKD patients in this ever-growing renal community who constantly struggle to make sense of their disease. I have written this book for you, so you can dream a bigger dream. I want you to secure your best life possible, just like I did.

As an author I cannot choose my readers. I'd like to believe that your attraction to this book stems from your desire to *do something,* even though you've been told *there's nothing you can do.* Actually, there's plenty you can do if you start now, while you have time in your favor.

If I've caught you in time, and you're ready to stand tall and walk *before* your chronic illness, this book will transform your life. All you need to do is start thinking more proactively with your future in mind. You target is all about living a quality life worth living.

Whether you realize it or not, your future is in your hands. You have one of three choices standing before you right now. One of your options would be to accept your diagnosis as an excuse to do nothing. Another option would be to accept your diagnosis as an excuse to live your remaining years in fear, with your disease dictating your destiny. The third and best option, gives you permission to stand above the crowd, by *embracing* new wisdom and advocating for your best life possible.

Cheers To Your Best Life!

Risa Simon

TABLE OF CONTENTS

Foreword

It was a serendipitous event that led to my first encounter with Risa. She was a patient in our transplant program at Mayo Clinic in Arizona, where I was the Operations Manager responsible for overall management of the abdominal solid organ transplant programs, including the Living Kidney Donor Program—a cause I feel deeply passionate about both personally and professionally.

From the beginning, it was clear that Risa and I had a common interest in "pro-active" management for chronic kidney disease patients and in promoting living kidney donation. Our common interest grew into a shared purpose—and our "thought bubble" grew to read: *"We Can Do More!"* We agreed there was much work to be done—Risa in her world and me in mine.

Risa and I developed a friendship. We would meet occasionally to discuss CKD patients and life in general. Whenever I talked on too long about transplant-related matters, Risa didn't get a glazed look in her eyes like others would—rather, she responded with matched enthusiasm. I knew I had met one of my people in Risa.

Among the issues we discussed, the gap in information and education for chronic kidney disease patients regarding all available treatment options, remained the common headline to our gatherings. We heard from patients that the information they were provided was often unclear, incomplete or missing. Assumptions were being made by providers on behalf of patients that dialysis would be the treatment plan, rather

1

than giving patients the information and opportunity to explore transplant options.

We knew that assumptions like those could adversely alter the course of a CKD patient's life. We also knew from the data that a certain percentage of CKD patients are not eligible to be transplant candidates. However, it is also true that many CKD patients could write a different end to their story if they were just given the right information at the proper time.

As clinicians, we can educate on clinical details, pathophysiology, side effects of meds and other relevant clinical information about the disease a person has. However no one's health care team can speak to what it's like to be the patient. That sacred role is reserved for those who have walked a mile in those shoes.

This book is a first of its kind written by someone who has walked that mile. Risa has outlined a heartfelt response to the dilemma you may not have known you were facing. The book before you can be your ticket to freedom—the only missing ingredient is you.

Risa has invested in your future by graciously taking on the role of personal tour guide. There is no better role model or cheerleader for you on this journey than Risa. It is my hope that you will use the information provided to take control of your health so that you can live your best life now.

I had the privilege of witnessing the transformation of the author, Risa, on her journey to freedom—and was even allowed the opportunity to play a role. Not only do Risa and I share the same goal for you—to live your best possible life—we also share one set of kidneys.

That's right. On June 8, 2010, I became a living kidney donor by donating my left kidney to Risa. The surgeries occurred simultaneously. It was my team of physicians, nurses and technicians who either performed or assisted in this surgical miracle that allowed me to give new life to Risa.

It was an invaluable experience to be both an RN and Operations Administrator on the "other side" of our system. One of the most gratifying experiences in being a living kidney donor has been the opportunity to witness the recipient bounce back metabolically after transplant. To know that someone's life is improved as a direct result of a decision made by me—there are no words to describe the "feel good" that derives from that.

The opportunity to be a living kidney donor for Risa was *my* privilege. The perspective I now have for what it's like to be a patient calling into our center, to be cared for in my department or checked into our transplant wing—is invaluable.

Meeting Risa was perhaps one of the most fortunate and significant things that ever happened to me. As you meet her in this book, I believe you will find that to be true for yourself as well.

Blessings,

Melissa Blevins Bein

Melissa Blevins Bein, RN, MS

3

Introduction

If you are one of the 26 million Americans diagnosed with Chronic Kidney Disease (CKD) who would like a chance to change your fate—this book was written for you.

While I cannot offer you a miracle cure, the information contained in these pages has the power to dramatically improve the quality of your life. I know this to be true because it happened to me.

My journey began in my early twenties when I joined this ever-growing CKD community with my own diagnosis. From that point on, I observed my life like the beads of sand sifting through an hourglass.

The diagnosis hit me hard as I now had the same disease that had taken my father's life in his early forties and my father's mother before I was born. This insidious genetic disorder known as Polycystic Kidney Disease or *PKD* kept reappearing like a wound that wouldn't heal. It was relentless. It had already attacked two generations before me, and it was now oozing its way into mine.

Years after my diagnosis, my brother, who had been told he didn't have the disease when he was tested as an adolescent, received the shocking news that he in fact had it too. He was in his late-thirties at the time and was almost instantly put on dialysis. The thought of following in the footsteps of the family members who had walked this path before me literally terrified me. This was not the life I had imagined for anyone in my family, and it certainly was not the life I wanted for myself.

Fortunately, I was told it would be years before I might feel the full effects of this disease. Much like a young person who ignores saving for retirement, that verbal prescription basically encouraged me to ignore my inherited DNA for quite some time. Call it denial, ignorance or just plain stupidity—I was frozen in my own fear.

Doing anything more than that didn't seem to matter much, as I was told there wasn't anything I could do to improve or reverse my diagnosis. Some nephrologists even told me *not* to return until I was "sicker."

This was an odd predicament to be in. On one side of the coin, it was reassuring to know I wasn't "sick enough." Yet, on the other side of the coin, I feared what "sick enough" would be like, once I did find myself in that situation.

It felt like a train was chasing me, and while it appeared that I could push myself to stay ahead of the locomotive, I had no sense of direction. As a person who typically plans for events, this one threw me for a loop. I felt clueless and powerless. Perhaps this is what caused me to become an entrepreneur? My thinking was if I couldn't orchestrate my own outcome, then perhaps I could orchestrate other people's outcomes.

I became the founder, president—and CEO of my own management consulting and seminar company. I was responsible for everything, yet my key role was helping clients more efficiently care for their patients. I traveled the country speaking at state dental conventions and consulted in private practices nationwide. Business was thriving and life was good for over two decades. Then insomnia and hypertension crept into my life, escalating me into bouts of anxiety. It was as if my soul was body-snatched by fear.

It was not until I experienced a panic attack on stage that I began to see things differently. I became dizzy and confused, and nearly went down in front of a ballroom of attendees. Although I was able to keep myself upright and hide my terrified mind from the group, I could not ignore the indisputable truth that stood before me. The sleeping *CKD/PKD* giant had finally awakened. It was time to shift gears and reapply for a far more important job. The job of CEO for my own health—not just my business.

My first step was to embrace my fear and make it okay to feel vulnerable. I then took a closer look at my situation, while exploring all renal failure options. During this process I stumbled onto some unexpected information about dialysis and transplantation.

What I discovered will astound you. It certainly astounded me. My first epiphany occurred when I discovered the truth behind dialysis. I had no idea that dialysis *before* transplant held significant *dis*advantages— and that the treatment alone practically guaranteed hideous side effects. I also discovered dialysis held higher mortality rates.

My second epiphany underscored the value of living kidney donor transplants. Here's where I discovered the huge difference between living-donor and deceased-donor kidney transplants, and the superlative value of a preemptive kidney transplant (a transplant performed before the need for dialysis). I also discovered that an approved living kidney donor could end your life-threatening wait—and that a living donor's kidney could last up to twice as long!

I was grateful to discover these differences, yet nothing stunned me more than the realization that I hadn't heard this information before. I then realized if I wasn't getting this information, you probably weren't either! How could our doctors be withholding this information from us? Worse, why weren't they teaching us to become more proactive patients? There is far more discussion about dialysis and vein-mapping, with little, if any, encouragement to explore transplant opportunities.

I was immensely frustrated by this model, and I felt compelled to do something about it. But the real tipping point didn't occur until I attended a *PKD* convention in the summer of 2008. At the time my renal function had dropped to 29%. I was drawn to the track on living kidney donor transplants, even though I had succumbed to the thought of *Peritoneal Dialysis* prior to attending this event.

The presenter, a handsome and articulate transplant surgeon with a charming French accent, filled the room with a bright light of hope. I was on the edge of my seat listening to each and every word as I studied his slides. He was revealing what no one else was talking about. Quality of life, improved outcomes, early referral and the value of preemptive transplantation. The information seeped through my veins with a palpable sensation of renewed vitality. The more I listened to his message, the more I realized just how much I had lost my way. Yet, as I gasped at the thought of letting myself get so far off course, it suddenly felt like I was "home."

I walked away from that meeting knowing I could do more. It was as if I was called upon to use my professional experience to make a difference for all those in need. I pledged to refocus my 25 year dental consulting and speaking career *into* helping renal patients and their healthcare providers achieve better outcomes.

Soon you will see a new opportunity standing before you too. The question for you is, what will you do with it? I know this is a bold new paradigm that takes courage and passion. Yet, I can't think of better traits to learn as you proactively plan to secure your best life.

If you are fearful about your future, know that your fear is a normal response to a chronic illness diagnosis. You are not alone. Over 26 million *CKD* patients stand in your shoes. Let the words of wisdom imprinted on these pages speak to your heart. Flirt with the principles, play with the philosophy and recognize it's time to start discerning what *is* in your best interest, and what *is not*.

Of course, this book is not just about the words you are reading. While the words hold great value and are critically important, it will be your understanding of the words and your unwavering commitment to shift from your old ways of *re*-acting to a new behavioral model of *pro*-acting, that will matter most.

If you've been told not to worry now because you have lots of time, start asking braver questions, like *"Time for what? Time to get sicker so I'll become dialysis dependent some day?"* The wiser question to ask would be *"What can I do now to shift my fate?"*

If your healthcare team truly understood the challenges you'd be facing, they would not be telling you that you have time. Instead, they would be encouraging you to *learn* more and *do* more to optimize your choices. Do not fall prey to the *Fistula-First* initiative—until you have thoroughly explored the *TransplantFirst®* movement.

Start by taking a fresh look at the power behind the proactive approaches in the pages that follow. Once you uncover the incomparable advantage in living donor kidney transplants, there will be no turning back. Of course, uncovering these advantages is one thing; doing the work is quite another.

Currently, there are tens of thousands of people waiting on a national kidney transplant list where your name will be added, if it isn't there already. Once you're on the list, you have to wait years and years before a deceased organ donor's kidney becomes available for you. This reality ought to be your most compelling reason to investigate *preemptive* living kidney donor transplantation as your first choice.

Once you discover the incredible benefits that preemptive transplants from living kidney donors can offer, you'll wonder why anyone would choose to wait idly when they could be doing so much more.

In this book you'll be able to fill your own *PEBO®* Toolbox, with systems specifically designed to help you *Proactively Empower your Best Outcome*. One of the most powerful tools you'll discover is the *Donor Magnet®* system. This revolutionary system is designed to help you position yourself as a deserving and desirable potential kidney transplant recipient. With a slight shift of mindset, these tools will give your story wings, so it can be heard by a greater number of potential living kidney donors who can help you.

I know this to be true because the *Donor Magnet®* system helped me attract over 21 offers in an 18 month period—and over half of them were from people I didn't even know. Of those offers, only six were approved for testing. Of those who were approved, only four fully tested. The fifth partially tested and the sixth changed her mind.

Of the four who fully tested, one retested because she was certain there was a mistake. No such luck for either one of us. Only one of the four qualified to be my donor.

Oddly enough, I'm blood type "O" which makes me a "universal donor," meaning I can give to *anyone*. You would think that *anyone* could give to me, right? Wrong. Universal blood type "O" donors can *only* receive from their own kind. In other words, blood type "O" can only receive from a blood type "O." This narrowed my playing field.

Another kidney conundrum occurred when I received an offer from a more suitable donor, while another potential donor was already testing on my behalf. Most centers only allow one potential donor to be tested at a time. I found myself sending mixed messages by accepting multiple offers. The problem arose when a potential donor called in to the center only to be told they're not needed because *someone else* was testing for me at that time. (*Be mindful that this can be the perfect formula for losing a potential donor!*) These are the types of roadblocks that you need to be prepared for with a "work around" in mind. More importantly, your potential donors need directive from you, so they are communicating updates as often as they have them. Being open, informative and communicative at all times will help all parties involved mitigate issues.

Because the donor qualification process can be grueling (and the challenge to find a suitable donor can take several weeks to several months—and even years for some), early engagement is essential. Oftentimes, the hardest part of this process is not so much in the doing or proactive planning. It's in the waiting and watching to see what blooms from all the seeds you planted.

Emotions intensify when a potential donor, who said they would call in— didn't; or worse, when you receive a call from your nurse coordinator stating that your most promising prospect was just disqualified.

It's important to realize that this is not an eleventh hour process. That is, unless you don't mind staring at a dialysis machine while contemplating your situation. I don't mean to sound harsh, but I am trying to jolt you out of that *"let's get sicker first"* trance that most of us tend to fall into because we believe we have more "time." If you wait much longer, it may already be too late to shift your fate. The bumps in the road that you'll most likely experience are far more manageable when you have time to repave your path. That's not the reality of kidney disease.

If you have the foresight to value your life as it deserves to be valued, you'll soon see this information in this book as an opportunity to extend and enhance your quality of life. This book isn't like one of those trains in pursuit of stealing your soul. It's merely a *life-whistle* blowing, prompting you to wake up and take action.

That *life-whistle* is precisely what triggered my relentless pursuit for a transplant. I did this by positioning transplant as my first and best choice. I can proudly say I was able to secure my best choice – first, without the need for dialysis.

The strategies and success stories shared in this book are now being provided to you. My goal is to help you secure your best choice (a transplant) – first, just like I did, without requiring dialysis beforehand.

While this book is not intended to replace sound medical advice, it does communicate an undeniable truth. A truth you rarely find in any doctor's office. It's the truth about how being a proactive kidney patient can open doors to unparalleled opportunities. You will be led through those doors while reading this book. You'll also be introduced to concepts designed to ignite your potential to secure your best outcome.

There is only one caveat for those who wish to get the most out of this book. You must be fully committed and willing to do the work in *advance* of urgent need. I implore you to ignore that inner dialogue that often cycles your mind like a lonesome cowboy song. Those all too familiar lyrics, *"I'm just not sick enough to think about this yet,"* are brainwashing you to believe something that couldn't be further from the truth. If you wait until you are *sick enough,* it may already be too late to *shift* your fate.

Fortunately, I was lucky enough to figure that out when I still had a chance to *shift my fate.* It took some work, and a lot of time, but boy did it payoff. I'm now living my best life ever. If I caught you in time and you're willing to do the work, this book can teach you how to live your best life too.

Even if you're reading this book a bit late in the game and find yourself already on dialysis, it's not too late to take advantage of our donor outreach *action steps.* You'll also gain insights on how to share your story and invite potential living kidney donors to lean in your direction. The key here is to get going *before* your health declines and squelches all hope for a transplant.

I often wonder what my life would be like if I hadn't attended that patient conference in 2008. Ironically, that day hit me as hard as the day I received this devastating diagnosis. This time, however, the news was profoundly uplifting. It felt liberated in a way I had never experienced before.

As that feeling came over me with a sense of peace and calm, I rightfully re-claimed a sense of control over my future by flipping the switch on my life's hopeless trajectory.

I started visualizing all the things I could do and all the possibilities in the road head. I could now see the promising fork in the road, rather than a cliff at the end of this troubled journey. It was then that I realized I never actually lost control of my life. I merely lived my life as if I did.

Attending that conference was not a coincidence. It was a blessing. Having this book in your hands right now is not a coincidence either. It is my hope it will be a blessing for you as well.

It is with profound gratitude that I am able to say I'm a *preemptive* (live-donor) kidney transplant recipient in excellent health. I honor this outcome as an *earned* blessing, achieved by my steadfast desire to learn more, do more and secure my best life possible.

Each day I wake with tremendous joy and appreciation for this extraordinary life I now live. Best of all, I'm free of dialysis. I've never been on it – and I hope to never need it.

This is what I want for you.

" I Was Seldom Able To See An
Opportunity Until It Had Ceased
To Be One."

– Mark Twain

Chapter 1: Now Is The Time!

Don't Let Your Diagnosis Dictate Your Outcome

I have no doubt that when you were diagnosed with Chronic Kidney Disease (CKD), you did everything asked of you. You changed your diet and upped your exercise game. And when you were asked to inspect food labels for sodium and phosphorous, you were as vigilant as a forensic investigator.

At least that's what I did, and a whole lot more. I became a devoted health fanatic. I was willing to do whatever it took to slow the progression of my disease. I gave up red meat, worked out as often as I could and restricted my foods to lean chicken and fish, grains and plant-based foods.

I also monitored my blood pressure, or rather I checked it obsessively. But my blood pressure would elevate from the mere thought of checking it, and each time I did, an even higher reading preceded the first. I felt like a cat chasing its own tail.

For the most part though, I felt pretty good about what I was doing to slow the progression of my disease. Yet even though I was doing many things right, I failed to examine the most important issue: *Was I doing enough?*

Are you doing enough?

What I mean is, are you doing enough to shift your fate and secure your *best life* possible? Until you

15

open your eyes to what someday could be the inevitable, you may never know the answer.

I am not trying to frighten you. I am trying to rattle your thinking though. I want this information to cause you to shift, so you will insist upon knowing more about what you can do before you've lost significant renal function.

> I had failed to examine the most important issue. Was I doing enough?

You simply cannot wait until you reach the point of needing dialysis to start working on a plan. The time to start planning is now. Set your plan in motion while you are still healthy enough to grasp the significant differences between your choices. Be *All In* and dedicate yourself to a daily process to secure your best outcome.

While I am fairly certain you already know what dialysis is, and how a kidney transplant differs, I want you to think deeper and wider about the difference between these two options.

Don't let the labels or their names disguise the way in which each one will affect your life. You can easily be fooled into thinking that you already know everything there is to know. Or perhaps you are stuck in a holding pattern, on a "need to know" basis. Believe me, you need to know!

When you don't have all the particulars, it is easy to think that you have more time than you actually have. This is an illusion. Give yourself permission to do your own investigation. If you are reading this and have never experienced dialysis, I encourage you to interview dialysis patients. You'll be amazed to learn first-hand what being a dialysis patient is really like.

16

Yet there are more serious issues to consider. Did you know that a realistic expectation for renal function from dialysis, is only 10 to 13 percent of what a normal functioning kidney provides? Did you also know that dialysis patients have extraordinarily high mortality rates—and that their risk of death increases the longer they're on dialysis? Evidently, nearly half of these dialysis-associated deaths are caused by cardiovascular disease—27 percent of which are caused by sudden cardiac death.

If your nephrologist would recommend dialysis when you approach 15% function, then ask yourself what you'd be gaining from this type of therapy? You don't have to be a rocket scientist to conclude that dialysis merely sustains the lowest level of function needed to keep you alive—but at what risk?

Who would consciously choose this therapy if a superior option was available? Your goal to improve your health must not be overshadowed by the delusions of this misrepresented equivalent.

I'm outraged that more CKD patients don't know the behind the scenes difference between dialysis and having a transplant. It almost feels as though these lost facts are a form of *"Don't Ask, Don't Tell;"* except most of us don't even know what to ask!

This concerns me and it should concern you too. As CKD patients we need to stand up and command the kind of outrage that other patient populations do. We can start by demanding that the risks and benefits of each treatment modality be more explicit. Our voices must be heard to ensure dialysis is not our doctor's first line of renal replacement therapy, particularly when the superior choice of a *preemptive transplant* has *not* been considered, discussed or proactively encouraged.

In this book you'll not only be exposed to undisclosed and rarely discussed

> **Our voices must be heard to ensure dialysis is not our doctor's first line of renal replacement therapy.**

information, you'll find tools and systems to instantly improve your chances of obtaining a better outcome.

I ask that you put on your detective cap and get out your magnifying glass before you get to work. There are unspoken differences between dialysis and transplantation, and you need to discover them now — before it is too late.

Most CKD patients fall short here, but you don't have to fall short. You can make a decision today by bridging the knowledge gap. I was able to turn myself around, and you can too.

Do not let your fear of the unknown scare you away from a better life. The fear that you sense is an illusion coming from the man behind the curtain who is making you think it is not safe to go there. Expose this *unwise Wizard* by recognizing that you have the freedom to become your own best advocate.

YOU: The Missing Link

Even though your healthcare team may not be encouraging you to plan for your future, there is a lot *you* can do without their permission or approval. It all begins by consciously choosing to be a champion rather than a victim. You can be the *strongest* link in the chain when you put your mind to it. You have the power to change your destiny — but it must begin with you.

Don't wait to hit rock bottom to make this important. By then it will be too late. The "Someday I will get this going" procrastination theory will get you nowhere fast. Start taking small steps right now. These small steps have the potential to lead to big time rewards.

Start by waking up each day with the mantra: *"I'm All In,"* and you will, at the very least, start each day more energized to make each day be the best that it can be. This self-directed journey will take you beyond what you may have already learned from your doctor's office *Dialysis and Transplant 101* training.

When you choose to become more engaged and knowledgeable, your world expands through your access to infinite wisdom. This journey will help you uncover hidden gems and avoid the landmines that no one is telling you about. You'll also be able to spot all the warning signs like *stop, yield* and *detour* here. These insights will help you build the type of courage that will compel you to speak up and be heard.

You will also be able to spot an odd sequence of events and then question the rationale of their sequencing to ensure they are in your best interest. For instance, when a fistula is being discussed without preemptive transplant dialogues preceding it, you'll know something is off. You'll discover that working towards bypassing dialysis, in favor of a superior option, requires advanced planning and a voice. Your voice.

Research show that only 2.5% of CKD patients received a kidney transplant as their first modality of treatment. A pathetic number that needs to change. You have the power to increase those percentages by simply refusing to sleepwalk your way to dialysis.

We must make kidney transplantation a primary therapy focus for ESRD patients—well before the need for dialysis has been identified.

Things You Need To Know

Are you aware of our nation's life-threatening organ shortage? Did you know there are over 90,000 people on the national kidney transplant waiting list? Did you know the average wait is four and a half years for a deceased-organ donor's kidney, and in some states like California and New York, it can be double that?

Can you imagine how that delay could force you onto dialysis—or even worse, cause you to get sicker while on dialysis? And did you know that as a patient gets sicker while they wait, they are often removed from the list because they no longer qualify for a transplant? Nineteen hundred people are removed from the list every year due to advanced illness and another 4400 people are removed due to death. That's 17 tragedies a day. Please, don't end up being one of them!

You won't be, if you consider and plan the option of finding a living kidney donor. A living kidney donor could *end your wait* all together. Such an option, as you will soon see, has unparalleled benefits.

Among the most remarkable, kidneys from living donors start working almost immediately once connected to the recipient on the operating table—and they can offer nearly double the years of function when compared to a deceased donor kidney.

Of course when considering a transplant from a living kidney donor, you'll need to find your own living kidney donor. Identifying and attracting potential living kidney donors takes time. Lots of time.

20

Living kidney donors won't offer to be tested for you until they learn more about your need. They also need to know the scope of what their involvement means, so that they can contemplate the significance of their selfless contribution.

Once a potential donor steps forward, it is best that they discuss their intentions with their family *(See Chapter 11)*, before calling into the transplant center for the initial telephone interview. If they pass the telephone screening, they will be scheduled for a battery of tests to see if they can be your donor. Then comes the waiting game from the transplant center's Selection Committee.

In the introduction of this book I explained how I experienced a number of donor related delays and disappointments. I urge you to be prepared for these types of delays. The goal here is to have a solid plan in place, but not without a donor backup. You'll also need a backup to your donor back up and so on.

Whatever you thought you were going to do or whatever you thought might happen *before* you started reading this book, will most likely change. That is, if you want to change your fate. The beauty of renewing your process now is that it allows you an opportunity to *test drive* these concepts in your mind *before* the only option left is dialysis.

Allow yourself the necessary time that you'll need to discover your best path so you can find your *groove*. Before long, all your hard work and preparation will fall into place like an engineered key sliding perfectly into its crafted slot, ready at a moment's notice to unlock your potential.

Step Aside From Your Past

Having a genetic kidney disease caused me to think as though I knew more than I knew. After all, I had observed family members suffering from the disease. What more was there to know?

Before my dad died from complications with PKD, I never considered that there might have been a better path for him to follow. Of course back then, living kidney transplantation and improvements in immunosuppression were slow to come.

I watched my dad struggle on dialysis for years and then fight for his life to thwart post-transplant rejection. Sadly, he lost that battle at the young age of 43. Years later, my brother started developing symptoms and was forced onto dialysis. He then waited on the list for a deceased organ donor's kidney for more than three years before he received his transplant.

When my brother was nearing the end of his transplanted kidney's term, he and his wife started discussing her possible involvement. Unfortunately, his immunosuppression threw a few wildcards into their plans with a couple of life-threatening setbacks.

This all began when my brother acquired a serious staph infection, which led to his hospitalization. His situation worsened before it improved, which put a huge strain on his heart and what remained of his transplanted kidney. This caused him to return for triple bypass surgery. After surgery he become dialysis dependent once again, yet this time he was on in-center hemodialysis.

While he was recovering, his loving wife Kim started making plans to be tested. During this time they discovered they were not only blood type compatible, they matched as well as if they were brother and sister! After months and months of testing and then more testing and delays, the news was announced. Kim was approved to be his donor. Our entire family was so relieved and deeply moved by the enormity of her selfless spirit.

I recall planning my trip to UCLA to witness this exciting event. It was by far one of the most memorable days of my life. I chose to walk to the hospital on that beautiful spring morning from my nearby hotel. There was something special in the air that day; something untold but felt. My surroundings were full of color, and the sound of traffic seemed so distant.

A hummingbird fluttered her wings before me as if she was trying to get my attention. And that she did. I stopped to admire her drink from a nearby bush of blossoms. As she sipped her sweet nectar, she paused momentarily to grace me with her presence once again. She danced about my face for several moments as if she was trying to tell me something. It was as if she was confirming a miracle was about to take place. Her presence and the promise of her message did not let me down.

Indeed, a miracle did take place that day—a gift of life. Yet this one was particularly special as it occurred while the donor was still living. It was as if my Kim gave birth that day. I guess you could say she did, only this time it was to one of her kidneys.

My mother and I were the first to visit her. She was up, eating and smiling—eager to hear how my brother was doing. Upon receipt of the good news, she ordered more food, as if it was a birthday party celebration.

In her pain I could see Kim's spirit rise above it all with pride and honor. She was a hero that day. And she will always be a hero to my family. Her incredible act of human kindness was by far the most loving thing we had ever witnessed.

Next, we were off to see my brother. Upon entering his room, I immediately noticed the improvement in his skin color. As he peered my way after taking hold of his hand, I called his name. I could also see an improvement in the clarity of his eyes. It was as if he was a new person.

Upon recognizing my voice, his eyes opened wider. He smiled with the sweetest smile. I instantly knew he was communicating so much more. He squeezed my hand so tightly that my rings left marks.

He had come through the operation strong as ever. My apprehensions dissipated; we began to talk. His first words were "How is Kim?" Relieved to discover that she was fine, he drifted off to sleep. The smile remained on his face the entire time.

What a gift it was for me to witness this event. It was like a sneak preview of the blessing I would someday experience myself. The education I got that day was better than any *Ivy League* college could ever teach me. It was so surreal.

After my brother's transplant, it was hard to even imagine I had considered dialysis as my first choice— even if only briefly. Although I became a believer from that point on, it did not instantly rid me of those worrisome thoughts that I had developed over the years.

That took time. Just as a distressed daughter cannot forget how her father struggled for years before his early death, I could not instantly stop my worries over this disease.

Looking Fear in the Face

Facing the worries remaining in the shadows of my mind wasn't easy. I knew I had to "up" my game. These worrisome thoughts were like a pesky gopher that would rear his head just when I thought he was gone for good. But then I realized, I could distract myself from all my worry by simply reaching out to help others. I was unconsciously transforming those pesky creatures into tri-colored rainbows of "feel-good," and I liked how it felt. I guess I was drawn to the process because I thought it was the right thing to do. Honestly, I had no idea it would be so rewarding.

Mostly, my worries centered on my labs. I was living from poke to poke, focused solely on the numbers and the phlebotomists that could be more sympathetic to my rolling veins. The challenge of the draw, however, paled in comparison to my requests for my results. You would think I had asked the CIA for a classified document. I even had to go so far as to impersonate an employee from my doctor's office so that the lab would fax me a copy. I couldn't believe I went to such measures just to get what was rightfully mine. I often wondered how many other CKD patients had to go through this. Or worse, how many patients even knew to ask.

Are you asking for a copy of your lab results?

I believe all blood draw laboratories should be *required* to give the patient a copy of their labs as soon as the results are in. Your doctor's office should also help you interpret the results so that they mean something to you. When you know your numbers and what they mean, you can use this information to your advantage.

You can also help your healthcare team recognize levels that are out of line—at the time it is recognized, so that immediate action can be taken. Don't wait until your next appointment for someone else to inform you. Be more accountable and take it upon yourself to do the work.

If you have not yet been educated on how to read your labs, insist that your doctor or nurse teach you how. Do not chance that everything will be caught by your healthcare professionals, or that the timing of their discovery will best serve you. They have a lot of patients besides you. Other patient results are already bombarding their fax machines. Don't get lost in the shuffle, or stuck at the bottom of the stack.

Of course there are issues attached to the knowing of these numbers, and I would be remiss to ignore the emotional side of this equation. While knowing your numbers is important, they can trick you into thinking you have tons of time—or conversely, scare you into believing death is imminent. Both exaggerations can wreak havoc on your emotions which can cause deviations to your game plan.

My emotions are still connected to my lab results and I can trigger those emotions in a moment's notice by imagining the sound of a fax coming through. If important renal numbers were stable, I'd give off a sigh of relief. If numbers worsened, a feeling of panic overcame me and stayed with me up until my next lab draw.

I eventually found a way to douse my anxiety through work distractions and through my husband's emotionally intelligent support. The diversions came to a screeching halt, however, when I was forty-nine years old.

That was the year when my numbers stumbled down a mountain like a lopsided boulder. They would slide down a bit, and then be anchored by some unknown force. Here they remained stable, but just for a while. It didn't take long before they shifted south again.

It was time to admit my disease was progressing. It was also time to get more serious about my future options. It was time work a better plan.

By age fifty-two, it was apparent that my plan to dodge the *full* effects of my disease had failed. I could now see that *I* was in part responsible for holding myself back. It was time to get real and make some changes.

The first thing I did was to shift my thinking from *I can beat this thing* to a more realistic view of approaching end-stage renal disease (*ESRD*) and renal failure.

Next, I threw out all my false beliefs—like thinking I knew the difference between dialysis and transplant or that I might never need either one of them. I had to recognize that my knowledge base was limited to the mechanics of these procedures and that renal failure was a very strong possibility in my future.

What I was lacking was evidence-based studies, patient feedback and viewpoints illustrating risks and benefits of one over the other. I'm not sure why it took me so long to become an *inquiring mind*. I guess I felt that if I was lacking information, or not totally comprehending the scope of my situation, my nephrologist would have told me so.

Nonetheless, I took it upon myself to begin my own exploratory journey. I realized if I wanted more answers I would have to find them on my own. And that's exactly what I did. Follow along, so you can do the same.

Life-Changing Wisdom Tips

1. Ask yourself if you are doing enough to secure your best life possible.

2. Insist on getting a copy of your labs and learn how to read them. Know your numbers and what they mean. Track your disease progression and hold your doctors accountable.

3. Be willing to see what your choices are with end stage renal failure—well before you need to make these choices.

4. Refuse the "Get Sicker First Plan." It is not in your best interest!

5. Become an inquiring mind. Learn as much as you can— then learn some more. Never stop learning.

6. Understand the real differences between dialysis and transplant, and the superlative benefits gained in preemptive kidney transplantation.

7. Educate yourself on the planning and procedures of living donor transplants.

8. Recognize that your best path will take time. Act early, come out ahead and you will never look back.

9. Use this life-changing wisdom to shift your fate—and prepare to live your best life!

"The Ultimate Authority
Must Always Rest With
The Individual's Own Reason
And Critical Analysis."

–Dalai Lama

Chapter 2: Taking Ownership

From that point on, it didn't take much for me to realize how vulnerable I had become. I had been depending on others to lead the way and by doing so, I had lost both time and opportunity. With only myself to blame, it became clear to me that I was the one who needed to create a better plan.

The first few steps after making that decision came rather easy to me. I took full ownership in developing a proactive plan, much like I took ownership in my own business. I had a mission and a vision, yet I knew I needed to learn more to make those purpose-filled statements count. I outlined the process and committed to doing the work necessary to achieve the best outcome.

Just having a plan of action was all I really needed to get going. I was like a high-powered vacuum, set to cover all ground. All I had to do was engage in the path before me.

My expectations became more realistic when visiting the nephrologist. While my visits had been geared to the discussion of labs, medications and the physical exam for the most part, I always created a window to discuss a bit more. Though my appointments were strictly for clarification and not for full-on education or philosophical exchanges, I was hopeful that they could become more of a mentoring session someday.

31

The one fortunate thing about my appointments was that my nephrologist was very knowledgeable and competent. He enjoyed explaining things to me. And while at times we disagreed, he always listened to my point of view.

He was also very generous with his time. He never appeared rushed. Of course the flip side was I'd often wait well beyond my appointment time before he made it to the room, but it was always worth the wait.

Yet, I still felt I wasn't getting all of the information I needed. I was desperately seeking more insight and I needed to be encouraged to really explore treatment options *in advance* of need. It was like being in the backseat of a car that was accelerating with no one at the wheel. I wanted to be driving my plan, with a GPS pointing to my ideal destination.

I yearned for an opportunity to *shift my fate*. Fortuitously, this quest of mine led me to a transformative convention in Dallas, Texas in the summer of 2008. It was a national meeting put on by the PKD Foundation. They had a number of tracks available to attendees, and one in particular caught my eye. It was a course on renal transplantation from living kidney donors.

Speakers included a transplant surgeon, a recipient and a transplant nephrologist. They revealed studies demonstrating improved outcomes from preemptive kidney transplantation while underscoring the risks associated with dialysis.

Suddenly, it was like the brightest light had been turned on in the darkest room. One by one, their messages unraveled the bandage I had unconsciously wound around my wounded heart. I felt like I had just won the lottery full of life-saving information. I was on fire and couldn't wait to get back to put those thoughts into action.

The entire experience spun my mind around like the blades on an automatic mixer, and by the time I returned home I was twirling even more. I knew I was on to something, and I felt that something was BIG.

I was stunned that I hadn't heard this information before. Then I started to wonder how many CKD patients were just as unaware as I was. As a CKD patient you deserve to know everything you need to know to make informed decisions. Yet, how would you acquire this information if it was not provided by the experts following your care?

It was like a black hole in the universe. Were healthcare professionals aware of this void? And if they became aware of it, would they consider filling this need in-house or by outsourcing it so that their patients could make informed decisions to improve their outcome for a better quality of life?

Unsure of the answer, I decided to become a part of the solution. I started to shift my two decade plus speaking and consulting career from the dental profession to the renal community. In doing so, I was approached by the Polycystic Kidney Foundation to head their Phoenix Chapter. I was also given an opportunity to become one of the National Kidney Foundation's PEERS program mentors, while continuing my coaching services to others. I spoke to renal groups and my transplant center about re-inventing patient education modules. It was as if I fortuitously found my perfect niche.

So here's the question I pose to you: "Are you ready to become a part of the solution too?" I invite you to try it on for size by simply flirting with the idea of becoming more proactive. No one is going to give YOU your best life. Not even this book without your participation. This book can only *assist* you in setting up and executing your plan. The plan, however, can only be developed and carried out by YOU.

Since no one knows what you want more than you do, what better person to be at the helm? You are the one who will keep your goals front and center at all times, not the busy doctor's office who's managing dozens of patients daily. There is a better way to fully participate in this quest to obtain your best possible life, and it all begins with YOU.

YOU: Your Body's CEO

Oddly enough, most of us don't realize that we are the CEO of our own body. Are you confused by that statement? Allow me to break it down. As an adult, you are in charge of what you eat, when you wake and when you go to sleep, right? Don't you choose the clothes you wear, how you style your hair, and how you engage in relationships—or not? Of course you do. You also decide what you are going to do each day, where you are going to go and the routes that will take you there. Of course you have responsibilities and commitments that direct your decisions, but you are the one who makes those decisions. You are your body's CEO.

If you're your own CEO, then why aren't you optimizing your power, like a CEO would, to ensure the future? It's okay to be *job sharing* with your healthcare team; in fact it is essential. I'm just encouraging you not

34

to choose the path that appears to have the easiest route—that is, dialysis—without researching other, more beneficial options first.

You cannot afford to be near-sighted here. You must be thinking about today, tomorrow and the rest of your life from here on out. Once you make your mind up that your life matters, you can start reclaiming ownership of your body and directing your future. Pledge to take yourself off *Automatic Patient-Pilot* or what I refer to as *APP®*. This promotion can be one of the most liberating things you will ever do.

But I'm Not Sick Enough Yet

If you're reluctant to go in any other direction than the one you are going in now *(because you think you are not sick enough yet, or because your doctor hasn't told you so)*, I implore you to snap out of it. You have fallen into a *CKD hypnotic stupor®*— and it is time to break free!

I've said it before and I'll say it again many times over: "Achieving your best life takes time. Lots of time." But isn't that true of everything that makes your life better? We spend a lot of time in school before securing a great job. We don't pick our husbands or wives without the effort to know them better. Children don't start talking right out of the womb.

Most things that are important to us take time to develop. And there is a lot of time and effort required in development.

It is no different here. If you think you don't have the time to do the work now, just wait and see how challenging it will be when your life depends on it.

The key is to not wait until you get sicker to start planning your future. Surely, you don't want to join the 350,000 patients in the U.S. who end up on dialysis, never knowing if they could have been transplant eligible?

Start taking *proactive* ownership in the possibility that you will most likely lose your remaining renal function someday. If, by chance, you live the rest of your life not needing to fully implement your plan, you can simply pass your wisdom on to others. You have nothing to lose but shame for not trying.

If you happen to be on dialysis already, waiting for a transplant, your goal is end your wait. Getting sicker will only keep you from achieving your goals.

The average wait on the national kidney transplant list is roughly four and a half years for a kidney from a deceased organ donor. In some regions of some states, like Los Angeles and New York, the wait can be more than double the average. Of course any length of time waiting increases your risk. Add multiple years of waiting and you're now compounding your risk.

The biggest risk while waiting occurs when your illness advances and health deteriorates. This can cause you to lose your transplant eligibility. If you're ineligible for a transplant, your life depends on dialysis. If you can't regain eligibility, you'll be on dialysis for life.

The key is to have a plan outside the deceased donor system. Taking on this new proactive approach can be a true game-changer in the fate of your future.

The Early Bird Catches The Worm

Start your journey before your disease progresses to a point of making tough decisions or to a state of urgency. If you don't want to "go there" until you feel you have to, I would suggest that you change your paradigm and start imagining that your need *is* now. Act *as if* your need is NOW!

Be willing to do whatever it takes to get into a proactive mode of thinking and planning. This strategy will keep you from emotionally charged *re-action* by moving you into deliberate and supportive *pro-action*.

The objective is to be so prepared that the process no longer involves you fretting over decisions. Instead, it will have you confirming your choices so you can make informed decisions *well before* you need to execute your plan.

Don't worry about how far out your future needs might appear to you now, or about the thought of ever needing renal replacement therapy. You don't have that crystal ball. What you need right now is *peace of mind,* knowing you have solid plan, if and when the need arises.

Action Follows Insight

Still not convinced? Keep reading. After all, you've just begun this exploration process and it's only Chapter 2. I have to confess that it took me quite some time to recognize the need. Give yourself permission to read on and learn more.

I have no doubt that you'll develop a thirst to learn more about the difference between dialysis and transplant, and as you do you will find yourself naturally transitioning into a more proactive and empowered patient.

The silver lining begins the moment you choose to enter this new path of discovery—providing you approach this process *before* you lose your power of choice.

> If, by chance, you live the rest of your life not needing to fully implement your plan, you can simply pass your wisdom on to others. You have nothing to lose but shame for not trying.

The ball is in your court.

YOU decide.

YOU decide if you want to navigate the best possible journey or sit back and ride the turbulent waves as they crash over your head.

It's not your nephrologist's responsibility, nor your husband's, wife's, child's, parent's or friend's. Only you can make a difference in this process by fully participating—starting right now. While loved ones can cheer for you and support you all the way, you are the one who needs to do the work. Take it from me. Better yet, take it from the number of highly enlightened proactive kidney patients who, like me, are now living their best life possible. *(Refer to testimonial stories at the end of this book).*

It's all about the timing and execution of your engagement. This is what will make all the difference in the world — your world, providing it's not too late and you're willing to do the work necessary to achieve your best outcome.

I truly believe this book didn't find you by accident. You were attracted to this book for a reason. I encourage you to see this process not as something that *might* make a difference, but rather as a golden opportunity that is certain to make *all* the difference in the world.

Life-Changing Wisdom Tips

1. Be accountable for your own health.

2. Plan to live the best life possible.

3. Don't expect to learn everything you need to know at the doctor's office.

4. Snap out of the CKD hypnotic stupor® you may have fallen into. You simply cannot afford to wait to get sick or any sicker than you already are.

5. Be willing to do the work.

6. Refuse to sit back and ride the turbulent waves of deteriorating health.

7. Start Early. Timing is everything.

8. Don't allow ignorant excuses to convince you that you have all the time in the world. You don't.

9. Use this life-changing wisdom to shift your fate—and prepare to live your best life!

" My Strength Lies Solely
In My Tenacity."

– Louis Pasteur

Chapter 3: Prolific Kidney Function

Now that you're energized to learn more, let's step back for a moment and take a closer look at the kidney itself. Weighing in at a mere half a pound each, these amazing bean-shaped organs are one of the most productive organs in your body.

Although most of us are born with two kidneys, healthy individuals need only one kidney to live a normal life. It's almost as if nature wanted to give healthy individuals an opportunity to donate one of their kidneys sometime during their lifetime.

Energizer Bunnies on Steroids

These bean shaped organs are often referred to as your body's master chemist, sharing layered levels of responsibility that outperform other organs by a mile. Your kidneys are the workhorses of your body. They have the extraordinary ability to filter roughly 200 quarts of fluid *every* 24 hours. That is over 50 gallons of fluid a day.

Can you imagine waking up each morning to 50 one-gallon milk cartons sitting on your kitchen counter?

> **Your kidneys are the workhorses of your body. They have the extraordinary ability to filter roughly 200 quarts of fluid every 24 hours.**

While you'd never be able to consume that much liquid in one day, your kidneys will be processing a similar amount of fluid before sunrise tomorrow.

Talk about being both energetic and resourceful. They're like Energizer Bunnies on steroids!

So What's Going On In There?

The primary function of the kidneys is to be much like our municipalities wastewater system. Just as a city's wastewater system treats and reuses wastewater, kidneys do the same for body fluids. As your kidneys sift through the 200 quarts of blood and waste fluid each day, they end up returning approximately 198 quarts of filtered fluid back into your blood supply. They hold back about two quarts of filtered fluid that they have identified as waste. That waste is then sent to your bladder, to be removed by you in the form of urine.

Fluid is classified as waste when it comes from the digestion of the foods we eat. Proteins like meat, fish, poultry or dairy products create the most waste, and they are the type of waste that only the kidney can filter.

Surprisingly, your kidneys are *not* usually used to breakdown sugars or starches. They only get involved when the glucose produced from those metabolic processes exceeds a normal healthy range for the body.

Under normal circumstances, the carbohydrates that we eat are broken down into water and carbon dioxide. However, when there is a surplus, your kidneys are called upon to eliminate the excess in the form of urine. When these signs show up as high glucose levels on your labs, it generally indicates a sign of diabetes.

Most of our organs have one main function. Take the heart for example. It is responsible for pumping blood throughout the body. Our lungs are responsible for oxygenating that blood and the pancreas is responsible for regulating the sugar level in your blood. The kidneys, however, are what you might call *overachievers*. They multitask several responsibilities at the same time.

For example, the kidneys are in charge of keeping our body balanced. Not symmetrically as you might imagine, although we do have one on each side. But rather by achieving and maintaining what is called *homeostasis*. Homeostasis is the process of maintaining the balance and stability of our body's *internal* environment.

As you might imagine, this is a multipurpose job, which can only be accomplished by combining several synergistic functions. Here is a list of those functions your kidneys perform to keep your body in balance:

- Balance the body's salt, potassium and acid content
- Produce hormones to stimulate red blood cells (*erythrocytes*)
- Control calcium metabolism and blood phosphates
- Regulate blood pressure
- Produce an active form of vitamin D
- Remove waste products, medications, and excess fluids

The Filtration Phenomena

Functioning like an all-night diner, your kidneys are taking orders and serving you 24/7. Each kidney, no larger than an adult's fist, has a filtration system with four-components to it, somewhat similar in concept to a residential water purification system.

A residential filtering process starts with a funnel into which the water flows into a membrane device within a chamber. Here the fluid is filtered as the liquid passes through. Then there is a transportation mechanism to move the filtered fluid towards its point of use and a collection reservoir to hold the filtered water until it's time to use it.

Now, take a look at how your kidney's filtering stages work:

1.   First, just as the residential water filtration process starts by funneling the water, our kidneys receive waste containing blood through the principal artery known as the *renal artery*.

2.   From there, the blood is moved through one of our kidneys many filtering devices (i.e., a membrane), known as *nephrons*. (Note that healthy kidneys have roughly a million functioning nephrons each. Each nephron is made of up three important components, the *glomerulus*, a *tubular system* and a *collecting duct*. This is important in the discussion below).

3.   When blood is exposed to the glomerulus, filtration is activated. The glomerulus is designed to provide a wide surface (membrane) for contact, so it can filter the fluid that flows by. The glomerulus is the master gatekeeper in this process. It intuitively holds back large particles which the body needs (like blood cells), and only permits small particles to pass through its membrane to be filtered.

4.   Once fluid is filtered through the glomerulus, it transforms into what is called *filtrate*. The filtrate then moves from the

45

glomerulus and enters the tubules and collecting ducts.

5. The tubules and collecting ducts determine if the fluid should be reabsorbed for your body's use, or be extracted as waste.

Tubules and collecting ducts are robust components of the glomerulus, in that they continue filtration while removing waste and reabsorbing essential nutrients and salts. Tubules aim to target the byproduct of protein metabolism called *urea*, with the goal of eliminating it.

Your tubules are attached to the glomerulus and loop through your kidney like a DNA chain.

Throughout this spiral loop, the tubules continue to process the filtrate, while allowing nearby capillaries to reabsorb salts, water and nutrients needed by your body.

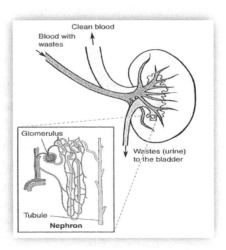

Useless waste is then sent to the bladder via the collection duct, in the form of urine.

As you can see, the entire filtration process includes the reabsorption of *good for your body* nutrients, while filtering and eliminating the *bad for your body* waste.

Hopefully, this more in-depth description of the role your kidneys play has given you a fresh perspective on how hard your kidneys have worked over the years and how important they are to your overall health. And though you may have already lost or will be losing more function, be grateful for what your kidneys have given you up to this point, and for what they are continuing to give you today.

A sense of gratitude has always been a powerful healing source for me. Even with the disease I inherited, I've been able to appreciate the hard work my kidneys provided for me for so many years.

If you've not done this before, I say try it on for size. You have nothing to lose and chances are, you'll feel a lot better. And you don't need to be a spiritual person, although that helps. Just be grateful for all that your kidneys have done for you throughout the years. Believe it or not, you'll make your kidneys happy just by doing so.

Your kidneys have worked hard in your honor. It is time to value their dedication and hard work. Speak to them silently, or aloud.

Don't worry if it seems foolish. This is important work. Tell them how sorry you are that you let them down (whether you are aware of something you might have done, or not) and promise to take better care of them from here on out. At the very least, you will be connecting to an energy that has never sensed support.

You might surprise yourself, as others have, by witnessing a slower progression in your disease.

Kidney Conundrums

Of course kidneys can only perform their job well when they are functioning at normal levels. Your kidneys most likely lack peak performance because something has caused their impairment.

There are a number of conditions that can cause renal failure. These include:

1. Chronic Pyelonephritis
2. Congenital Disease of the Kidney
3. Dysplasia
4. Glomerular diseases
5. Hypertensive Nephropathy
6. Interstitial Nephritis
7. Polycystic Kidney Disease (PKD)
8. Type I and II Diabetes

Even if you don't see your condition on the list, there's one thing you and many other CKD patients can count on. That is, diseased kidneys are relentless, in that they struggle to work at their full and intended capacity at all times. Yet, while struggling to give you their all, they are still functioning at a reduced level. They are like a marathon runner with the flu. No matter how hard that marathon runner may try to give the race their all, the runner is still functioning at a reduced level.

That is why they are unable to filter blood efficiently. Byproducts showing up in your blood and urine are signs that this is so. When those byproducts stay in the blood, problems occur.

Conversely, other products that are supposed to stay in the blood (like protein) end up causing problems by spilling out through your urine.

Yet even though your kidneys may not be functioning at their full and intended capacity at this time, they haven't given up entirely—and neither should you!

So whether you have diabetes, and can't convert glucose into usable energy, or hypertension with uncontrollable blood pressure or other kidney diseases that cause damage to the kidneys—it's time to make a choice:

> 1. You can continue a static mode at a snail's pace, by doing nothing other than what you are told to do until you get sicker, or

> 2. You can take on a more proactive role in your health starting right here, right now. All you need to do is pledge to be *"All In"* that is, if you'd like to slow the progression of your disease and design a plan to secure your best possible future.

> You can do this *before* knowing with absolute certainty what your needs will be. You will, however, have to fight off any thoughts that try to trick you into believing you're moving too fast.

The choice is up to you. Use this book to help you understand your choices better. This book is *not* intended to be a replacement for your professional healthcare advisers. Quite the contrary, actually. It was written to be used as a pocket-companion to help you fill in all those information voids, so you can ask important questions and become more informed and proactive.

Look to it to expand your awareness and build courage, or simply filter your thoughts more logically so you can challenge standard norms. Allow it to help you create your own *healthcare reform* so you can become more accountable as you partner with your nephrologist.

Simply refuse to let your body's inability to reverse your disease *sabotage* your ability to change your fate. You are the producer, choreographer and director of this movie. You were not intended to be the *stand-in*.

> **Even though your kidneys may not be functioning at their full and intended capacity at this time, they haven't given up entirely—and neither should you!**

Life-Changing Wisdom Tips

1. Your kidneys work hard for you: understand and respect what they do for you even at a reduced level.

2. Although most of us are born with two kidneys, healthy individuals need only one kidney to live a normal life.

3. Recognize that your kidneys, although small, are really powerful workhorses that perform more bodily functions than any other organ in the body.

4. Expand your awareness to filter your thoughts more logically so you can challenge standard norms.

5. Create your own healthcare reform by becoming more accountable for your own health, while partnering with your nephrologist.

6. Refuse to let your body's inability to reserve your disease sabotage your ability to achieve the best outcome. You deserve to live the best life possible.

7. Even with reduced function, your kidneys haven't given up entirely, and neither should you.

8. Use this life-changing wisdom to shift your fate—and prepare to live your best life!

" The Best Thing About The Future Is
That it Comes One
Day At a Time."

– *Abe Lincoln*

Chapter 4: Know Your Numbers

Learning Lab Language

By now you are probably aware of the key areas you need to monitor on your labs. For example, if you are diabetic, you are most likely watching your glucose (blood sugar) levels. If you are anemic, you are watching your iron levels and red blood cell markers like your hemoglobin and hematocrit, among a few others.

Depending on the condition of your kidneys or other health concerns you are monitoring, there could be a number of areas you'd need to keep your eyes on. Some of these tests can initially sound like an announcement on an international flight. You might be able to make out a few of the words, but you could never translate what it all means.

But if you are going to be *All In* with respect to your disease, then you must learn to speak the *lab language.*

Here are the three star performers you must get to know intimately:

1. **Glomerular Filtration Rate (GFR)**

    Your *Glomerular Filtration Rate,* or *GFR,* is the measurement of how efficiently your kidneys are filtering waste from your blood. Think back to what you just learned about kidney filtration. As discussed, the waste-filled blood enters the kidney through the renal artery, and then it intuitively passes through your kidney's nephrons to be filtered.

53

You may recall that each nephron has a filter, which is comprised of a *glomerulus*, a *tubular system* and a *collecting*

> **Your GFR number is a leading indicator of the progression of your kidney disease.**

duct. The role of the glomerulus' wide surface area is to come into contact with the fluid that flows by it, so that the fluid can be filtered.

When the glomerulus is not working well, it loses its ability to sift, sort, clean and recognize what needs to be held and sent back. How well the glomerulus is working is determined by the glomerulus filtration rate, or *GFR* line item on your lab results. Your GFR number is a leading indicator of the progression of your kidney disease. When your *GFR* is inadequately functioning (or filtering), this number will show below normal on your lab results.

The *GFR* of a healthy young person could be as high as 130, while a healthy person in their 70's should not be below a *GFR* of 75. As you can see, *GFR* declines with age, just as a car's air filter becomes less efficient after so many miles.

When *GFR* values fall below 60, that's an indication of Chronic Kidney Disease. When that level further declines to less than 15, the patient is considered to be in renal failure. Oftentimes a lab will just list your *GFR* as being >60 or >15, without providing actual numbers. If the lab you are using does not list your *GFR* as a standard measurement, you can calculate it on your own with a little help from a *GFR calculator* which can be found at the National Kidney Foundation's website link:

http://www.kidney.org/professionals/kdoqi/gfr_c alculator.cfm

All you need to do is enter is your age, race, gender —and your *serum creatinine* (which will be discussed next)— and the program will do the math for you within seconds. It's just that easy. And, best of all, it's free!

2. **Creatinine (*Cr*)**

   Creatinine, also known as *Cr*, is a specific type of waste product measurement in your blood. This test is run to gauge your kidney's ability to breakdown muscle cell waste. Healthy kidneys have no problem processing *Cr* out of the bloodstream as waste. That waste is then flushed out of the body in the form of urine. Conversely, when your kidneys are not functioning sufficiently, your body is unable to process the waste. When this happens, an excess of *Cr* builds up in the blood, causing this marker to rise.

   Your goal is to keep your *Cr* number within normal limits, which is typically in the range of 0.6-1.1.

3. **Blood Urea Nitrogen, (*BUN*)**

   Your Blood Urea Nitrogen, or *BUN* is the amount of *protein* in your blood and urine. Most likely when your blood showed a high level *BUN* and a

high level of *Cr*, and low estimated *GFR*, your
doctor recognized you had kidney disease.

In addition to these three star performers, here is a
sample list of some other important markers to observe:

1. **Hemoglobin:** Hemoglobin is the part of red blood
   cells that carries oxygen from your lungs to all
   parts of your body. Your hemoglobin level tells
   your doctor if you have anemia, which makes you
   feel tired. If you have anemia, you may need
   treatment with iron supplements or a hormone
   injection called erythropoietin (EPO). The goal of
   anemia treatment is to reach and maintain a
   hemoglobin level of at least 11 or 12.
2. **Hematocrit:** Your hematocrit is a measure of the
   red blood cells your body is making. A low
   hematocrit can mean you have anemia and need
   treatment with iron and EPO. You will feel less
   tired and have more energy when your
   hematocrit reaches at least 33 to 36 percent.
3. **TSAT and Serum Ferritin:** Your TSAT and serum
   ferritin are measures of iron in your body. Your
   TSAT should be above 20 percent and your serum
   ferritin should be above 100. These levels help
   you build red blood cells. Iron supplementation
   may be needed here.
4. **Parathyroid Hormone (PTH):** High levels of
   parathyroid hormone (PTH) may result from a
   poor balance of calcium and phosphorus in your
   body. This can cause bone disease.

   Ask your doctor if your PTH level is in the right

range. Your doctor may order a special prescription form of vitamin D to help lower your PTH.

5. **Calcium:** Calcium is a mineral that is important for strong bones. Ask your doctor what your calcium level should be. To help balance the amount of calcium in your blood, your doctor may ask you to take calcium supplements as well as a special prescription form of vitamin D.

6. **Phosphorus:** If your phosphorus levels are high, it can lead to weak bones. Your doctor may ask you to reduce your intake of foods that are high in phosphorus and take a phosphate binder with your meals and snacks.

7. **Potassium:** Potassium is a mineral in your blood that helps your heart and muscles work properly. A potassium level that is too high or too low may weaken muscles and change your heartbeat. Your dietitian can help you plan your diet to get the right amount of potassium.

8. **Urine Protein:** Protein in urine, as known as proteinuria or microalbuminuria, occurs when proteins are not properly processed by the kidney's filters. This causes protein in urine. Temporarily high levels of protein in urine can occur in younger people after exercise or during an illness. Protein in the urine discovered on a microalbumin test may often be the earliest sign of diabetic kidney damage. Persistent protein in the urine is often an early sign of chronic kidney disease.

9. **Serum Albumin:** This is the most abundant protein found in blood plasma. It is essential for maintaining osmotic pressure needed for proper distribution of body fluids between intravascular compartments and body tissues. It also acts as a plasma carrier. Too much serum albumin in the body can be harmful. Albumin protein can pass into the urine when the kidneys are damaged.

As you can see, there are a number of categories to get familiar with, and this list is only a partial snapshot of what may show up on your labs. Don't worry about memorizing all the names and definitions. Just get familiar with the value each one of them holds.

Blood Pressure & Body Weight

Of course you can't forget the two very important markers that you won't find in your lab report, such as your *blood pressure* and *body weight*.

Blood pressure plays a significant role in the progression of your disease. Frequent monitoring at home will assure you that your readings are consistent with the reading in your doctor's office.

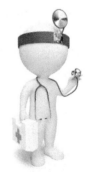

Blood pressure readings are only as good as the records you keep. You will have nothing to compare to—or report from, if you are not documenting your readings along with the date and time of day.

Use the *Blood Pressure Log* in the Forms and Chart section of this book. The goal here is to check your blood pressure at the same time of day to see if there are variances during those same periods.

If you are not monitoring your blood pressure on your own at home, you could be sabotaging an opportunity of slowing the progress of your disease. You could also be hindering your chance of reducing your cardiac risk factors, should your blood pressure get out of control.

Be sure to use a blood pressure monitor that has been calibrated with the one at your nephrologist's office. Simply bring your monitor in to your next appointment and tell your doctor or nurse that you would like to compare readings from your monitor to theirs. This failsafe method should be repeated every 6 months.

> **Be sure to use a blood pressure monitor that has been calibrated with the one at your nephrologist's office.**

Calibrating your monitor is simple. Simply start by taking the first reading with your own monitor and record your results. Use a piece of paper that has a line drawn down the middle so you can create two columns: one for your monitor readings and one for the doctor's office. Place your name above the left column and your doctor's name about the right column. Record your reading on the first line under your name.

Now, ask your doctor or nurse to follow with a reading from their monitor. Record those findings in the right column, adjacent to your first reading. Repeat readings in 15 minutes intervals, using both machines. Be sure to wait a few minutes between readings to give your arm a chance to recover.

If you find the readings are basically within the same range, or within just a couple of points of each other, then 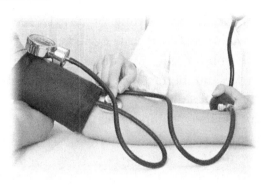 your monitor is accurately depicting readings conducive to your doctor's office readings. That is your goal.

If you find that your monitor is just a bit low or a bit high in comparison to your doctor's monitor, you can simply take that into consideration when recording and evaluating your home readings.

If, however, the readings appear to be several points apart, then it could be time to upgrade your monitor to a different brand or model, or time to assess your cuff size. I never realized that the wrong cuff size could throw your numbers off so much. It's true.

Take it from a person who was using the wrong cuff size for months and months before discovering why my home readings were significantly lower than my doctor's office readings. That factoid put all my presumptions about *White Coat Syndrome* into questionable review.

To check your cuff size, measure your arm with a tape measure just above your elbow. (It is best to follow the manufacturers' instructions for measurement, as they vary). Compare your size with the manufacturer's measurement range for the cuff that you own. If your cuff is too large or small for your arm, you should replace your cuff with one that is a more appropriate size.

If the model you own doesn't sell sized cuff replacements, you will want to purchase a new machine. When this is the case, be sure to find a manufacturer that provides a variety of cuff sizes and instructions for measuring your arm, in order to avoid repeating future issues.

While a good reading to shoot for would be 120/80, an even better reading would be 110/70. While I never witnessed readings that low before my transplant, my goal was simply to get my blood pressure down and keep it down by taking my blood pressure medication at the same time each day, and by reporting my findings to my nephrologist at every visit. This should be your goal as well.

If you take blood pressure medication, like most CKD patients do, you need to be certain that the medication you are taking is in fact doing what it was intended to do. Do not assume that since you take a prescription drug for your blood pressure, that it is working, or that it is still working after months or years of taking it. What may have worked earlier this year — or even last week, may not be as effective today. Often times, blood pressure management may require two or more synergistic medications to be effective.

As for your body weight, you need to watch fluctuations so that you can maintain it at a healthy level. A dietitian can suggest how to safely add or delete extra calories from your diet.

Talk to your doctor's renal dietician about weight changes so that they can be managed properly. It is also good to know your ideal Body Mass Index, or BMI. Your BMI is a number calculated from your weight and height. It does not measure body fat directly, but research shows that BMI correlates to direct measures of body fat, such as seen in underwater weighing.

BMI is used as a screening tool to identify possible weight problems for adults. Your BMI can be calculated by following a formula that divides your weight in pounds by height in inches squared, and then multiplying the result by a conversion factor of 703. Here is a link that will help you enter the numbers into a preset formula:

www.cdc.gov/healthyweight/assessing/bmi/adult_bmi/english_bmi_calculator/bmi_calculator.html

The Five Stages of Kidney Disease

Gaining a better understanding of each stage of chronic kidney disease will also help you gain insight on how fast (or slow) your disease is progressing, and it will help you measure the effectiveness of the protocols you are currently following.

Insights related to your level of kidney disease can also give you a better understanding of what stage your disease is in. This comprehensive snapshot below will help you determine your current level of CKD, which will give you a benchmark for monitoring the progression of your disease moving forward.

To help you better understand CKD levels, we will use the National Kidney Foundation's (*NKF*) guidelines of the five stages of Chronic Kidney Disease.

These stages use your *GFR* rate as the universal measuring tool.

NKF's Five Stages of CKD:

Stage 1:   **Normal *or* high GFR (GFR > 90 ml/min)**
Stage 1 CKD represents kidney damage with a GFR at a normal or high level of function, greater than 90 ml/min. There are usually no symptoms to indicate the kidneys are damaged. Because kidneys do a good job even when they're not functioning at 100%, most people will not know they have Stage 1 CKD. If they do find out they are in Stage 1, it is usually because they were being tested for another condition, such as diabetes or high blood pressure (the two leading causes of kidney disease). It is not until they discover a higher than normal level of *Cr* or *BUN* in blood work, or blood or protein in the urine, that suspicions arise.

Stage 2:   **Mild CKD (GFR = 60-89 ml/min)**
Stage 2 CKD is kidney damage with a mild decrease in GFR, resulting in a GFR of 60-89 ml/min. There are usually no symptoms to indicate the kidneys are damaged. Because kidneys do a good job even when they are not functioning at 100%, most people do not know they have Stage 2 CKD. This is usually discovered

when running tests for another condition, such as seen in Stage 1, like diabetes or high blood pressure.

Stage 3:   **Moderate CKD (GFR = 30-59 ml/min)**
Stage 3 CKD is kidney damage with a moderate decrease in GFR, resulting in a GFR from 30-59 ml/min. As kidney function declines, waste products build up in the blood causing a condition known as "uremia." In Stage 3 you are more likely to develop complications of kidney disease such as high blood pressure, anemia (a shortage of red blood cells) and/or early bone disease. Symptoms include fatigue, fluid retention, urination changes, kidney pain, sleep problems, itchy skin, muscle cramps and/or restless legs.

Stage 4:   **Severe CKD (GFR = 15-29 ml/min)**
A person with Stage 4 CKD has advanced kidney damage with a severe decrease in their GFR, which has fallen to a range of 15-30 ml/min. If you have Stage 4 CKD, it is likely that you will need dialysis or a kidney transplant in the near future.

Stage 4 holds the same symptoms as listed in Stage 3, with the addition of nausea, taste changes, loss of appetite, difficulty concentrating, and nerve problems. In Stage 4, you are also likely to develop additional complications like heart disease and other cardiovascular diseases.

Stage 5: **End Stage CKD (GFR <15 ml/min)**
Stage 5 CKD is what is known as end stage renal disease (ESRD). This is when your GFR falls to a level of 15 ml/min or less. At this advanced stage of kidney disease, the kidneys have lost nearly all of their ability to do their job without help. This is when dialysis or a kidney transplant is needed to survive. Symptoms include those listed under Stage 4, with the addition of changes in skin color, making little or no urine, swelling of the eyes and ankles, tingling of hands and feet, and increased skin pigmentation.

For more information on the Five Stages of Kidney Disease, visit: http://www.nationalkidneycenter.org/chronic-kidney-disease/stages

Honor Your Kidneys

Checking your numbers should be like checking in on a best friend. When you honor and care for your kidney function as you would a best friend, you'll always keep your health front and center.

The most effective way to stay intimately acquainted with all of your numbers is by recording what you can at home. Keep a file for your blood

> When you honor and care for your kidney function as you would a best friend, you'll always keep your health front and center.

pressure readings and your labs. You can create a visual

65

chart to keep your eye on fluctuations by using an excel spreadsheet or graph paper, a pencil and a ruler.

All you need to do is record your blood pressure readings on one graph, and your lab results on another. (Use the *Lab Chart* and the *Blood Pressure Log* in the Forms and Chart section of this book). Having this information at your fingertips can be extremely helpful. And, while it can be frightening at times to see how numbers have shifted, there is nothing more frightening than discovering that you could have done something to improve your consequences if only you had known.

If nothing else, this recordkeeping exercise will allow you to emotionally process your thoughts and feelings before you see your doctor. And by doing so, you will have a more productive visit. This process helped me formulate important questions to ask my doctor, rather than be distracted with my emotions.

Most of all, this record keeping process will put you back in the driver's seat. It is time to say *bye-bye* to that old uninformed patient who was tempted by the demon of denial. This is about putting yourself on a more empowered platform. Here you can refuel your inner guide and enlist all your care providers to help you achieve your best life possible.

The days of waiting for others to pass on critical information are long gone for the Proactive Kidney Patient *PKP*. A *PKP* doesn't waste time waiting for others to tell them what's going on. They take ownership for their health because they value their life.

Mind you—this is not about you having to *go it alone*. It is about *partnering* with your healthcare professionals. Knowing your *GFR*, *Cr* and *BUN* will, at the very least, allow you to more effectively partner with your nephrologist. This partnership will inspire you to become more accountable and more proactive. As you become more aware and engaged, you invite your nephrologist to also become more engaged and accountable by supporting ideal clinical outcomes, long before the need for dialysis approaches.

Simply choose *not* to accept standard recommendations without filtering them for yourself. Think like a nephron. Use your brain to filter out all the potentially damaging information and keep only that which will serve your best health interests. You will be stronger for having done so.

Be mindful to examine what you believe to be potentially damaging before filtering it out, by having a meaningful discussion with your nephrologist. This will ensure that you truly understand the ramifications of your intended plan.

Sound decision-making is always backed by information and logic. Previously held justifications for *not wanting to know* must now be over-shadowed by the more important stuff. That stuff just happens to determine your ability or inability to attain your best possible life.

Life-Changing Wisdom Tips

1. Learn to speak the lab language and know what your key markers are and what they mean. Become intimately familiar with your GFR, CR and BUN.

2. Chart your labs from each draw by using the *Lab Chart* in the Charts & Forms Section of this book. Compare findings to your previous lab results to ensure that you are aware when and to what level your numbers change.

3. Calibrate your home blood pressure machine with your nephrologist's office and be certain you are using a properly sized cuff to ensure accuracy. Record your blood pressure reading using the *Blood Pressure Log* in the Charts and Forms section of this book.

4. Work with a renal dietician to keep your labs and weight under control.

5. Familiarize yourself with the Five Stages of CKD. Monitor your progression by using its associated GFR scale so you will always know where you stand.

6. Create a partnership with your nephrologist and their support team in an effort to build a trusting relationship that serves your best future.

7. Use this life-changing wisdom to shift your fate—and prepare to live your best life!

"We Ourselves Feel That What
We Are Doing Is Just A Drop In The Ocean.
But The Ocean Would Be Less
Because of That Missing Drop."

-Mother Teresa

Chapter 5: Awareness, Awakenings & Realities

Body Awareness

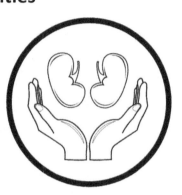

You probably never thought much about being consciously aware of your body. After all, the body tends to let you know when it needs your attention. If you are still able to fit into your favorite jeans, or if you've been feeling something for so long that you've become numb to the signals, you may be oblivious to certain signs and symptoms.

It's like not realizing there is a strange noise in your car's engine because the radio's turned up too loud. Having the radio drown out the engine noise doesn't mean that everything is ok with the engine. By the same token, a lack of pain—or chronic, ongoing pain, which your body has accepted as normal, doesn't mean that everything is okay there either.

Developing an awareness of your body and the energy that flows through it can be quite helpful. It can help you identify new symptoms and describe what you are experiencing.

How do you become more aware of your body you might ask? The answer is simple. Just pause periodically to become more mindful and less distracted with extraneous surroundings, just as you might stop to reflect on the day's events before saying *"Good night"* and turning out the light.

Test it out right now. Pretend you are at a stop light waiting for it to turn green. Use the delay to *pause* for body awareness. Start by straightening your spine. While bringing your chest up, take a long deep breath in.

Now, exhale slowly with the intention of relaxing your neck and shoulders. As you breathe in and out, pay particular attention to any tension you may hold in specific areas of your body.

Once identified, imagine the light just turned green. Now give yourself permission to *let go* of that tension as you exhale. You can incorporate this relaxation technique while driving. Just be sure to follow the actual light signals to guide you, as opposed to your imagination of color changes. As you awaken your body and tune in to its needs, you will find peace in the process of letting go.

This can help you recognize common CKD symptoms that you should be discussing with your doctor. These symptoms include:

> **As you awaken your body and tune in to its needs, you will find peace in the process of letting go.**

- High *or* uncontrolled blood pressure
- Nausea and vomiting
- Poor appetite
- Trouble sleeping
- Anemia & weakness
- Fatigue or inadequate energy
- Dry, itchy skin
- Muscle cramps

- Frequent urination
- Pain or difficulty urinating
- Puffy eyes
- Fluid retention: hand and feet edema

While these symptoms are common in CKD patients, they can also be symptomatic of other diseases. They can also reveal to the doctor important information about how your disease is progressing. Because of this, your doctors must be made aware of your symptoms, and to do that, you must be aware of what you are experiencing so that you can report it. Your doctors can only help you if you are making them aware of what you need help with.

Thinking that your symptoms aren't that important, or simply forgetting to mention them, could be like leaving out the one piece of evidence that could help your doctor solve the mystery behind your pain and discomfort.

Often times, a simple diet or medication change can resolve a specific situation, or at least prevent it from getting worse. Minor changes might also eliminate symptoms all together.

Signs and symptoms are often your body's way of crying out for help: "Hey! Pay attention to me! I don't like being ignored. Please notice the signals I'm giving you before you cause irreparable damage!"

Ignoring signs and symptoms can be more dangerous to your health than ignoring the Surgeon General's warning on a pack of cigarettes.

What makes this so? Your symptoms are warning you about something that has already manifested. It is not just a caution statement regarding a potential risk. It's already occurring.

As you pay closer attention to your body and its signals, record your discoveries. You can do this with a dedicated log. (Use the *Body Awareness Log* in the Forms and Charts section of this book). This will help you evaluate trends so you can identify harmful behaviors.

You can stop mindless damage by recognizing what isn't working well for you. All you have to do is recognize it and then make a conscious effort to shift gears.

Just imagine yourself back at the stop light:

1. Pause at the red light for body awareness.

2. Straighten your spine.

3. While bringing your chest up, take a long deep breath in.

4. Exhale slowly with the intention of relaxing your neck and shoulders.

5. As you breathe in and out, pay particular attention to any tension you may be holding in specific areas of your body.

6. After you have identified the tension or discomfort, try to determine what is causing the pain.

7. Now, imagine the light turning green.

8. Let the green "go" light help you to *let go* of all tension and behaviors that may be causing it on each exhale.

9. Now shift gears by embracing new behaviors to mitigate recurrences.

10. Record your symptoms and share them with your doctor at your next visit. If symptoms are of a more urgent nature, then call your doctor's office immediately.

How Can I Slow The Progression?

The National Kidney Foundation suggests several ways to potentially slow the progression of kidney disease. Here are just a few keepers:

- The use of "ACE Inhibitors" to control blood pressure. *ACE inhibitors have also been found to help protect kidney function.*

- Work with a renal dietitian to:

  - prevent or control diabetes.
  - prevent or lower protein in your diet.
  - restrict sodium in your diet.
  - restrict phosphorous in your diet.

- Stay physically fit. Exercise 30 minutes a day, three or more times a week.

Exercise helps most people to improve muscle function, lower blood pressure and cholesterol, and maintain a healthy body weight.

▪ Avoid taking pain-relieving medicines, especially non-steroidal anti-inflammatory drugs known as NSAIDs, (such Advil or Motrin) as they are known to be kidney toxic even with short-term use and liver toxic with long term use.

▪ Drink six to eight glasses of water each day, particularly if you are taking pain-relieving medicines.

The objective here is to slow the progression of your disease by doing as much as you can to keep your kidneys strong and healthy.

Side-View Mirror Approach

Don't wait to get sick (or sicker) to decide what your next move is. Think like the statement on your car's side-view mirror: "Objects in the mirror may be closer than they appear." Now, imagine that the words say:

"Renal Failure May Be Closer Than it Appears!"

Don't be like the drug addict who waits to hit rock bottom before getting help. Instead, be proactively focused on your bottom line rights:

1. You have the *right* to live the best life possible.
2. You have the *right* to feel as good as you possibly can.

75

3. You have the *right* to educate yourself.
4. You have the *right* to make informed decisions.
5. You have the *right* to seek better options.
6. You have the *right* to share your story and advocate on behalf of yourself and millions of others, without shame.

There is no shame in self-advocacy, as it increases awareness for all those in need. There is, however, shame in ignoring opportunity. In fact, there is more than shame. There can be deep regret, like the regret that a bear might feel after walking into a bear-trap. Prevent yourself from falling into such a trap as well while you still can.

Remember your side-view mirror—*Renal failure could be closer than it appears.* Like a Boy Scout—Be prepared. Whether you believe this is important now or not, you have nothing to lose by simply preparing yourself for the best outcome possible.

It's not a matter of *if* you believe you will ever develop complete renal failure, it's a matter of experiencing failure of a different kind. The failure to do something while you still could.

Consider teaming-up with your nephrologist to slow the progression of your disease, while proactively planning your best possible future.

> It's not a matter of if you believe you will ever develop complete renal failure, it's a matter of experiencing failure of a different kind.
> Failure to do something while you still could.

Not quite sure how to get teamed-up

with your doctor? Start by asking yourself these questions:

1. "Is my doctor a good *fit* for me? Do I feel a connection?"
If the answer is no, determine why you feel that way.

2. "Is there a sense of trust, or sincere interest in my health and wellbeing?" If the answer is no again, the wise thing to do is find another doctor.

If after changing doctors you still don't feel a connection, seek to find another until you do feel a connection. Your life will instantly appear better when you believe that your doctor genuinely cares about you and has your best interests in mind.

It's important to sense that you feel understood and that your doctor "gets" you! Without this feeling it's challenging to *team-up*.

Feeling understood is the perfect recipe for building respect

> **It's important to sense that you feel understood and that your doctor "gets" you!**

and trust. You deserve to have a doctor who cares about you and your future. Refuse to accept anything less.

I met with at least five nephrologists over the course of eight years. Sometimes I felt initial excitement or promise, like a good first date. But as is the case after many first dates, that feeling seemed to vanish over time as we would get to know one another better.

Be it busy schedules or just bad days, I had to trust my gut when it told me this physician was not a good fit for me.

Sure it takes bravado to switch doctors, and a lot of energy as well, but it was so worth it in the end. If you think your insurance plan will restrict you from switching, simply ask for a *second opinion*. Most good insurance plans will not deny you that privilege.

A solid relationship with your nephrologist and their medical support team will make all the difference in the world for you. At least it did for me. It allowed me to reveal more information, ask braver questions and enter into dialogues that I wouldn't have entered into otherwise.

You should be able to do the same. Your medical team is one of your most important links on this journey, but they are only as good as the relationship you have fostered with them. Exercise your freedom of choice. Then speak up and be heard.

Proactive Prerequisites

Being proactive isn't just about marching forward like a parade of soldiers. It is more about forward momentum, like a race car driver shifting to get into first position. It is fueled by passion, purpose, strategic planning and intention. It doesn't hurt to have an optimistic belief system either; in fact it may very well turbo charge your outcome, as it did for me. Keep in mind that likes attract likes. You have nothing to lose by believing that all things are possible. At the very least, it will draw you closer to your dreams.

When you operate from this position, your decision-making process will become more intuitive, like knowing which way to turn at the next corner, or selecting the best route to your destination. This perception will allow you to feel in control of your destiny. One of my favorite quotes is: *"Luck is What Happens When Preparation Meets Opportunity."*

This statement suggests that it is all about preparation. Preparation leads to opportunity. Opportunity leads to perfect timing. Perfect timing leads to optimal results, or what some would refer to as luck.

> **Preparation leads to opportunity. Opportunity leads to perfect timing. Perfect timing leads to optimal results, or what some would refer to as luck.**

How do you ignite this perpetual motion? By focusing on your intentions, not your fears. Focus on what's in your best interest and work a plan to get there. Don't let inertia slow you down any more than it already has.

Develop a hunger and a thirst for learning as much as you can so that you can make decisions that matter most. Act as if you don't know anything about chronic kidney disease. Then, reexamine it all as if you were learning it for the first time. You may be surprised to find that you had an incorrect perception about one aspect or another regarding your chronic kidney disease or its end stage options.

Once you rectify these erroneous thoughts, you can reengage with laser-like focus on a fresh slate.

CKD in America

According to the National Kidney Foundation 26 million people in the U.S. have CKD. That number suggests that one in nine American adults are affected. More alarmingly, 90% of the 26 million people affected don't even know they have the disease. To add insult to injury, an additional 20 million people are *unaware* they are at an increased risk for developing CKD.

Since CKD can often progress for years undetected, until it has advanced into more noticeable and irreversible stages, preventive measures have been challenging at best. Then, to become dialysis

> 90% of the 26 million people affected with CKD don't even know they have the disease, and an additional 20 million people are unaware they are at an increased risk for developing CKD.

dependent without years of planning or contemplation is like being separated from your family and deported to another country all at the same time. You never know what hit you and you hope that you'll awaken from this bad dream real soon.

Most patients who are transplant eligible think they can just get on the list and receive a transplant relatively soon. They don't realize that the supply of donated organs cannot meet the demands of our population.

Let's take a closer look at this life-threatening crisis we have experienced for years in America.

Deceased Donation: An Alarming Reality

Even though 2.5 million people die in the U.S. every year, only 15,000 of those deaths represent consented organ donors. Of those donors, only one-third qualify after further evaluation. This is where the donor's health history, or the trauma which caused the death, disqualifies the organ(s). What does that mean?

It means that in a country which needs over 90,000 kidneys and growing, we need at least 45,000 deceased donors with two good kidneys.

With only 5,000 deceased organ donors a year, that leaves 85,000 (at the time of this book's publication) without, and waiting for years for their name to be called. Clearly, the call to correct the disparity in our nation's organ crisis requires a supply beyond deceased donation. This is where living donation comes into play.

Living Donation: A Promising Paradigm

When we combine deceased kidney donations with living kidney donation opportunities, the formula looks far more promising. For example, our country could *end the wait* all together if we just add one-third of the people in attendance in the Brickyard at the Indy 500 as qualified *living* kidney donors. And that doesn't include most of those seated infield!

Yet, the vast majority of people haven't realized that they actually have two kidneys— and that a healthy person can live just as well with *one* kidney as they can with *two*. Moreover, few people understand that a kidney donor's remaining kidney expands as if it functioned at the power of two.

81

Living kidney donors are courageous, selfless individuals who want to make a difference. Read their stories in the *Donors & Recipients Tell Their Story Section* of this book. Their journeys are both inspiring and thought provoking.

Their insights and intentions have changed my world perspective, and I am certain they will change yours too. If nothing else, they will take your breath away.

My living kidney donor renewed my life, saved me from dialysis and allowed me to regain my health beyond my wildest imagination. A true blessing that I honor every day.

Life-Changing Wisdom Tips

1. Develop an awareness of your body. Document your symptoms and the sensations you are feeling in your Body Awareness Log so that you can report them to your doctor.

2. Use the "**side-view mirror**" to recognize that your renal failure may be closer than it appears.

3. Find a doctor that you respect, trust and connect with. Do not settle for less.

4. Focus on your intentions, not your fears. Keep your eye on what's in your best interest and commit to work a plan to get there.

5. Recognize that the nation has an organ shortage and seek to understand how living kidney donation saves lives.

6. Open your mind and your heart to living kidney donor stories and the prospect of what it would be like to receive the gift from a living kidney donor. *(Refer to Donors & Recipients Tell Their Story).*

7. Use this life-changing wisdom to shift your fate—and prepare to live your best life!

" If You Don't Know Where
You Are Going, How Can You Expect To
Get There?"

– *Basil S. Walsh*

Chapter 6: Critical Crossroads

Few people are diagnosed during the early stages of kidney disease, so it's likely that you may not have been diagnosed until your disease was in its more advanced stages. Due to the late timing of diagnosis, the need for dialysis and kidney transplants around the world continues to grow.

Johns Hopkins estimates the need for Americans currently on dialysis to jump from over 400,000 to 2 million by year 2030, due in part to the rising rates of diabetes. Combine that with the ever-growing number of ESRD patients (>90,000 at the time of this book's publication) who are waiting on a list for a kidney transplant and the numbers become even more frightening.

With a running average of about 16,000 kidney transplants performed in the U.S. annually from both deceased and living kidney donors, it's easy to understand why countless lives are lost while waiting. Dozens of names are removed from the list daily—and *not* because they were granted a kidney for their transplant—but because their body could no longer survive the wait.

YOU cannot afford to walk this slow and uncertain path. The stakes are too high. Your goal is to think bigger and

> With a running average of about 16,000 kidney transplants performed in the U.S. annually from both deceased and living kidney donors, it's easy to understand how countless lives are lost while waiting.

brighter—long before you know you are in urgent need.

While the most common tendency is to hold off on planning events until there is more certainty of need, this concept is a bit different. It's like starting a fund for your children's college. You don't know if they even want to go to college, or if they'd be accepted. Yet, you don't stop planning, dreaming and preparing to give them the best life possible. As the quote underscores:

> "**Luck** is what happens when **preparation**
> meets **opportunity**."-*Elmer Letterman*

This viewpoint impelled me to do the necessary work in advance of unknown need. I now hold immense pride and appreciation for my proactive diligence—a diligence that transformed me into the luckiest girl alive! When you plan for unpredictable events in your life like I did, you'll be positioning yourself (and your luck) to attract limitless possibilities. Yet, if you wait until you are more certain that you'll need to do this work, you'll most likely find yourself scrambling, with limited options.

Dialysis or Transplant?

To make a decision between dialysis and transplant, you must first understand all sides of each option along with their respective risk-reward ratios.

Let's start by taking a more detailed and descriptive look at dialysis. *Dialysis* is the mechanical process that attempts to mimic a percentage of your body's natural kidney filtering process. Dialysis may be your only *lifeline* if you have been told you're transplant ineligible. Yet, most people don't realize there's a preferred choice or that they could be eligible for a transplant instead.

What I found most surprising is that dialysis only replaces a small percentage of kidney function. A realistic expectation for dialysis is about 10-13 percent of what a functioning kidney provides. Dialysis cannot regulate levels of fluids and minerals, nor does it produce erythropoietin or 1,25-dihydroxycholecalciferol (calcitriol), as part of the endocrine system. Though it is an invaluable lifeline when transplant is *not* an option. In fact, it is the only option to filter waste

> **Most people don't realize that dialysis only replaces a small percentage of kidney function.**

for transplant ineligible patients who require renal replacement therapy. The question for those who do have a choice is "How long can dialysis sustain my life—and what type of life would I be living?"

The type of dialysis might also influence your decision. There are two types of dialysis, *peritoneal dialysis* and *hemodialysis,* and while you may already be somewhat familiar with dialysis, let's take a closer look.

Peritoneal Dialysis

In peritoneal dialysis, or *PD*, dialysis is performed inside the cavity walls of your abdomen. Inside the cavity, there is a membrane lining called the peritoneum. During PD, a mixture of dextrose (sugar, salt and other minerals) is dissolved in water. This dialysis solution can only enter your abdomen by way of a pre-surgically placed catheter that has both in-flow and out-flow connectors.

If you are considering PD, a specialist will need to determine if you'd be a good candidate before proceeding. Contraindications could be a hernia, space restrictions or muscle weakness in the walls of your abdomen. The surgery for the *PD* catheter is often performed laparoscopically, under general anesthesia.

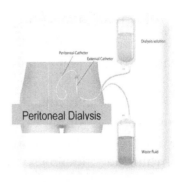

Peritoneal Dialysis

The catheter is a soft, flexible plastic tube about the length of a ruler and the width of a pencil. One end of the catheter is placed into the peritoneal cavity and the rest of the catheter will come through the patient's lower abdomen, underneath and to the side of the belly button. It exits the body through a very small opening called the exit site.

Often times the patient can be discharged the same day of surgery, but sometimes they will need to be kept overnight for observation.

The exit site is monitored by a PD nurse to observe proper healing and to ensure there are no problems with the catheter. Most patients need to wait at least two weeks after surgery to begin PD dialysis.

The *PD* procedure begins by connecting the catheter to a gravity feed IV bag of special dialysis solution. The solution is designed to attract waste products and extra body fluids through a process that is similar to static electricity.

At the completion of the procedure, a cauldron of waste products exit the body through the outflow connector into an empty gravity feed PD bag. Initially, the process is very proficient when fresh solution enters the abdomen, yet as more waste combines with the solution, the process becomes less efficient. And while a higher concentration of dextrose could be considered to increase efficiency, it can be of great concern to diabetics or patients dealing with weight issues.

Each cycle of draining and refilling is called an exchange. After each exchange, the solution must remain in the abdomen until the next exchange. This is called dwell time, and it can make the patient extremely uncomfortable or self-conscious from the extra weight being carried around in their abdomen.

Peritoneal Dialysis offers two options. They are referred to as:

1. Continuous Ambulatory Peritoneal Dialysis (CAPD), and
2. Continuous Cycler-assisted Peritoneal dialysis (CCPD)

With CAPD, a fresh bag of dialysis solution is gravity fed through the catheter into the abdomen and after 4 to 6 hours of dwell time, the waste filled solution is drained into the bag. The cycle is then repeated with a fresh bag of solution and the process continues. There is no machine required. The entire process is accomplished by gravity. The new solution bags are hung at a level above the abdomen, and the empty bags for draining are placed at a level below the abdomen to assist with gravity flow.

There are usually three to four exchanges during the day, with one long dwell time overnight while sleeping. As you can imagine, this can be an extremely time intensive process which takes some getting used to.

It is also important to consider what it would be like to have extra fluid and weight in the abdomen, in addition to the challenge of securing a clean and private place to do the exchanges. Self-discipline is essential here, as users must remember when to do the exchanges and be willing to set aside the time for each exchange. Multiple exchanges need to be performed each day — every day. There are no days off. Be certain this is what you want before selecting this option over other options, particularly if you are transplant eligible.

If time is your main concern, another option can be consider in *PD* dialysis. This option uses a continuous cycler called Continuous Cycler-assisted Peritoneal Dialysis (CCPD).

With CCPD, a machine is used to fill and empty the abdomen, three to five times during the night while you sleep. (For light sleepers who have trouble falling asleep and staying asleep, this could be an issue).

Each morning upon waking, the fluid from the last exchange during the night, remains in the abdomen all day. While not required, it is often best that the patient does at least one more exchange around mid-afternoon, to increase the amount of waste removed. This extra exchange also prevents excessive absorption of fluid.

Hemodialysis Dialysis

Now let's move to **hemodialysis.** In hemodialysis, the blood circulates outside the patient's body and moves through a hemodialysis machine's special filters before returning to the patient.

Hemodialysis requires access through your blood vessels in order to connect to the machine. This access is called vascular access. The three types of access are:

1.   Arteriovenous(AV) fistula
2.   Arteriovenous (AV) graft
3.   Venous catheter

A fistula is a connection between any two parts of the body that are usually separate from one another, and would otherwise not be connected. In dialysis, an *AV fistula* is created by attaching a native artery to a vein in an extremity, such as the upper arm.

This allows the vein to mature by growing larger and stronger for repeated needle insertions. It also improves blood flow. It is believed that the an AV *fistula* is a better option than an AV *graft* or catheter, as it seems to provide the best blood flow with fewer complications.

An *AV graft* is considered when you have small veins that won't develop properly into a fistula from a direct connection. In this case, the vascular access is

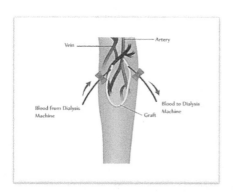

accomplished by connecting an artery to a vein using a synthetic tube, or *graft*, implanted under the skin in your arm. The graft then becomes an artificial vein that can be used for repeated needle placement.

A graft doesn't need time to develop like a fistula, so it can be used sooner after placement, often in less than 3 weeks.

A *Venous Catheter* is a tube inserted into a vein in your neck, chest or leg near the groin. The catheter has two chambers to allow a two-way flow of blood. No needles are required for this type of dialysis, making access more appealing to the patient. Yet, catheters are not ideal for permanent access as they can clog and are prone to infection. They can also cause narrowing of the veins in which they are placed.

Ideally, catheters are not used for more than a few weeks to a few months. Nephrologists will often give the *disapproving mother look* when they hear the word catheter, as they feel this access is far riskier than AV fistulas and grafts. For whatever it's worth, I have heard some pretty amazing stories about these so-called temporary devices. One CKD patient told me she used her catheter without incident for over 3 years, while waiting for her transplant, and my own brother had great success with his catheter for 9 months of use while waiting for his second living donor transplant.

All and all, catheters are intended only for patients who are suddenly diagnosed with renal failure or whose disease progressed so quickly that there is insufficient time to secure permanent vascular access before the need to start hemodialysis.

Surgical access for fistulas must be performed months *before* the need for dialysis, to allow time to form properly. Fistulas must also be checked to ensure proper function and efficiency, in order to minimize complications.

Keep in mind that long-term dialysis dependency requires the fistula to be used several times a week, for several hours at a time. With this type of repeated use, it is not uncommon to experience vascular access problems, including fistula malfunctions and thrombosis.

Sadly, these issues are the reason for over 25% of hospital admissions, in the dialysis population alone. It is believed that over 85% of patients on dialysis experience fistula malfunctions like, clotting, infections and failures throughout their dependence. Most failures are due to progressive narrowing of the surgical connection, or stenosis of a vein from trauma, which likely comes from repeated venipuncture during access for dialysis.

Understanding the process of hemodialysis is important before choosing dialysis. In AV fistula or AV graft dialysis, two needles are used — one to carry blood to the dialyzer and one to return the cleansed blood to your body. (There are specialized needles that allow two openings for two-way flow of blood, but these needles can be less efficient and can extend the time of each treatment).

There are several strategies for needle placement to mitigate problems with repeated sticks. However, it is your responsibility to keep the access site clean and free from trauma. Even the use of a blood pressure cuff can create problems on your access arm. It becomes your responsibility to speak up to prevent blood pressure readings on your access arm. It is also important to remember not to lift heavy objects with that arm, or wear tight clothes or jewelry. Likewise, you'll need to keep yourself from sleeping or leaning on your access arm.

There's no doubt that dialysis can and has saved lives. The question here is if you had the choice, would dialysis provide the quality of life you deserve?

When asked, dialysis patients often say the treatment itself can be debilitating, demoralizing, painful and extremely restrictive of their schedules. Whether they are tethered to a machine in an outpatient setting for hours a day, three times a week, *or* at home exchanging fluids several times a day, *every* day, this treatment option can be grueling.

Long-time users often regard dialysis as a treatment that's actually postponing their death, as opposed to a treatment that's preserving their life. That is why I want you to think long and hard about your choices, while you still have the luxury to choose.

So while it is not uncommon to think that dialysis isn't that bad; it isn't good if you could have had a kidney transplant instead.

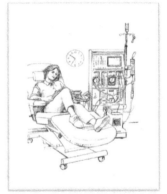

Sadly, a good number of dialysis patients never knew they would have qualified for transplant before dialysis.

It is believe that roughly 25% of all dialysis could still pursue transplant. The problem is they lack the knowledge and the skill to do so.

Why such a disconnect? Here's what's lacking:

1. Factual Comparisons (Dialysis /Transplant)
2. Superior Value In Preemptive Transplantation
3. Encouragement To Seek A Living Donor

In addition to a void in education, I also discovered that some renal patients were told they had to be on dialysis for one year before they can be considered for a transplant. Who is at fault here? The dialysis center, the referring nephrologist, the primary care doctor, clinics owned by dialysis centers—or transplant professionals who have an opportunity to educate their referral sources about the benefit of early transplantation, but don't?

Perhaps all of the above. And, while the Department of Health and Human Services, *HHS,* continues to insist that renal patients be informed about transplantation, the lack of reimbursement for time spent counseling only provokes non-compliance.

The most significant incentive to do the right thing comes from the *Centers for Medicare and Medicaid Services, CMS, 2008 ESRD Conditions for Coverage.* This payment-based persuasion mandates that dialysis facilities educate patients about transplantation, within 45 days of the initiation of dialysis, in order to get payment on billings. This mandate was put into place to ensure patients understood the value of having a transplant.

One way CMS hoped to enforce this requirement was through the use of their ESRD Conditions for Coverage Form 2728(5), which requires answers to questions like, "Has the patient been informed of their kidney transplant options?" If not, why not (i.e., medically unfit, patient declined). Hence, the center is reminded that a stipulation of coverage goes beyond the treatment they provided.

Yet, if education is not provided until the patient is in the dialysis center, isn't it too late? One can argue that it is always "better late than never," and that should be the exception, not the rule. Nephrologists need to offer a series of transplant exploration discussions *long before* dialysis is even being considered. In my mind, putting off patient education about transplantation—until the patient is dialysis dependent—is an unconscionable practice which is in desperate need of change.

Of course, renal transplantation is not for everyone, because not everyone can qualify as a candidate, or maintain their health status while waiting on dialysis for a qualified donor. Yet they all deserve the information before this superior option is taken away.

> If you believe you could be a candidate for renal transplantation, now is the time to understand the ramifications of choosing dialysis over transplant, as you may never get this opportunity again.

If you believe you could be a candidate for a renal transplantation, now is the time to understand the ramifications of choosing dialysis over transplant, as you may never get this opportunity again. Take advantage of the timing to learn more—starting today.

A Kidney Transplant

A kidney transplant is one of the most common transplant operations in the U.S. The procedure involves putting the donor's kidney, which has been skillfully separated from their body, into the recipient's body, so that it functions like the recipient's own kidneys once functioned.

The procedure is performed under general anesthesia, while you are completely asleep and pain-free. A Foley catheter is inserted into the bladder.

Typically, the native kidneys are left in place unless they are causing problems with infections or are too big for the space available. The reason for this is to minimize surgical morbidities or the urgent need for dialysis should a problem arise.

I, on the other hand, had enlarged kidneys taking up the bulk of the real estate within my small frame. It was as if my disease represented too many houses and hotels on my abdominal *Monopoly* board. Because of this, a decision was made to remove them at the same time as the transplant surgery.

Their parting was a doubly sweet bonus, because I was allowed to donate my kidneys to PKD research. Since they were no longer serving me, they could now be used to help find a cure for others who suffer from this disease. And while my offering pales in comparison to the heroic magnitude of a living kidney donor's gift to a CKD patient in need, it gave me a *peek-a-boo* glimpse at what it might feel like to give an organ to a greater cause.

You might be surprised to learn that the new kidney is not placed near the recipient's existing kidneys. Instead, it is typically placed on the right side of the pelvis in a location referred to as the iliac fossa. This location offers a wider choice of arteries and veins for reconstruction. Sometimes, and for various reasons like space considerations, the kidney is placed on the left side.

That's what happened in my case. My new kidney was placed on the left side (as shown below), due to my enlarged liver. I have an enlarged liver, which is not uncommon for *PKD* patients, known as polycystic liver disease, or *PLD*. Fortunately, in most *PLD* cases, patients rarely have liver function issues, even though the size of their liver increases considerably.

My transplant surgeon, the legendary Dr. David C. Mulligan at Mayo Clinic, Arizona, was well versed on my particular situation. This is why he chose to place my new kidney on the left side, even though it was a far greater challenge for him to do so. His goal was to give my enlarged liver, which is on the right side, more space. I cannot begin to tell you how thankful I am that he had the foresight and the expertise to do so.

Whether the new kidney is placed on the right or left side, its renal artery is connected to the *external iliac artery* and the renal vein of the new kidney is connected to the *external iliac vein.*

Transplanted Kidney Location

Once these two vessels are saturated, they are unclamped and the new kidney plumps up and turns pinkish. This process occurs from the recipient's own blood supply.

The next hope is to see urine start to form and pass through the new kidney's ureter, which is the tube that carries urine to the bladder. At this point, the ureter has not be connected to your bladder.

As soon as urine is observed passing through the ureter, the transplanted organ is considered a success. The "flow" observed is often referred to as *Golden Champagne*. Fittingly, a moment of mindful applause acknowledges this remarkable victory.

Next, the ureter is prepared for attachment to the urinary bladder. This is done by attaching the ureter to the mucosa in your bladder muscle. A stent or plastic tube is often placed through the ureter across the attachment to help the healing and mitigate potential flow restriction.

The stent must remain in place for a set amount of weeks after surgery for proper function and healing. The stent can cause discomfort for some—myself included. Honestly, though, it was a minor inconvenience compared to the grand scheme of things. And believe me, the grand scheme was indeed grand!

Rest and Recovery

Most transplant patients are hospitalized for about four days and then closely monitored at home for a period of four to six weeks. During this time there are several visits a week for labs and clinic appointments to ensure your new kidney is functioning properly. Theses visits also support your recovering, as your transplant team monitors how well you are adapting to your new life on immunosuppressive medications.

Life-Changing Wisdom Tips

1.   If you were considering dialysis before picking up this book, go back and evaluate how vascular access or abdominal catheter placement surgery is part of that deal which must be performed before dialysis can begin. Recognize that healing time is required and unexpected issues can delay the treatment.

2.   If you were considering dialysis before picking up this book, understand the side-effects associated with dialysis. Understand that dialysis can be debilitating, demoralizing, extremely restrictive—and often painful.

3.   If you were considering dialysis before picking up this book, understand the actual percentage of kidney function dialysis replaces. Ask yourself if that is what you hoped for?

4.   Understand what's involved in a kidney transplant procedure. Compare the difference of one surgery over ongoing dialysis treatments. The choice should be clear.

5.   Use this life-changing wisdom to shift your fate—and prepare to live your best life!

"Failure is Only The
Opportunity To More
Intelligently Begin Again."

– *Henry Ford*

Chapter 7: The Transplant Experience

The First Kidney Transplant

The *first cadaveric kidney* transplant was performed in the United States in 1950 on a 44-year-old woman named Ruth Tucker, who had PKD. Unfortunately, since immunosuppressive drugs had not yet been developed, her new kidney was rejected just 10 months following the transplant surgery.

Four years later, the first *living kidney donor* transplant was performed in Boston. The living donor and the recipient were identical twins in their twenties, Ronald and Richard Herrick. Ronald and Richard were both in the military serving their country at the time of the Korean War. Richard was suffering from nephritis near the close of his duty in the Coast Guard—so he was sent to a hospital in Massachusetts to be close to his family. Soon his illness advanced into renal failure. His older brother Van, sister Virginia and twin Ronald asked doctors about donating one of their kidneys in order to save their brother's life. A decision was made that because Ronald was an identical twin, his kidney might be able to help save his brother's life. Surgery was scheduled to be performed on December 23, 1954 at the Peter Brigham Hospital by Dr. Joseph Murray.

What a Christmas present! As nearby radios played Bing Crosby's *White Christmas* and Bill Haley and The Comets' *Shake, Rattle and Roll*, this life-changing event went down in history as one of the best White Christmases ever, not only for the Herrick family but also for the future of all CKD patients.

Ronald was discharged after 14 days (a whopping 13 days more than my living kidney donor's hospital stay in 2010), and Richard was discharged in 37 days (which was 33 more hospital nights than my own post-transplant stay). As indicated by these recovery times alone, there have been significant medical advances made since that first live kidney donor transplant.

Ronald married and went on to teach at the University of Maine in Augusta. In 1997, he celebrated his 50th anniversary of that first transplant live kidney donor transplant.

Richard married Clare Herrick, the nursing supervisor who volunteered on that Christmas weekend to care for Richard. They had two children, one a teacher and the other became a dialysis nurse. Richard enjoyed good health before developing problems in his new kidney that were unrelated to the surgery. With his health failing, he died on March, 14, 1963, at home in Shrewsbury, MA, with Clare by his side.

From that point on, dozens of kidney transplants were performed, and the success rate continued strong among identical twins. One of those success stories involved Johanna Nightingale, another one of Dr. Murray's patients, who received a kidney from her twin sister at age 12 in 1960, at Peter Bent Brigham Hospital in Boston, MA.

On December 28, 2010 Johanna celebrated her 50th anniversary for being one of the longest surviving single kidney transplant recipients. Just another remarkable story that exemplifies why Dr. Murray won the Nobel Prize in 1990 for his discovery that a transplanted kidney, in the absence of immunosuppression, can function well under these conditions.

In 1964, immunosuppressive medication became available for preventing and treating acute rejection. Nearly a decade after Dr. Murray's groundbreaking kidney transplant, the first liver transplant followed. Then in 1967, the first heart transplant. Anti-rejection drugs have helped to boost surgery success tremendously.

Today, kidney transplants are considered one of the easiest and most successful of all organs to transplant.

Transplant Evaluation

Choosing transplant over dialysis requires transplant center pre-approval. Of course, you can't get approved until you've been tested, and you can't be tested until you've been referred for evaluation. That is typically initiated by your nephrologist.

It's important to encourage your nephrologist to refer you for transplant evaluation as early as possible, preferably around 25 GFR. That will allow sufficient time for donor testing. You should also do your homework to decide which center you would like to be referred to.

The best way to determine this is by discovering what kidney transplant centers are in your area, or near your preferred location(s), and by assessing their respective transplant volume and success rates.

> It's important to encourage your nephrologist to refer you for transplant evaluation as early as possible.

Once you have been referred, you will receive a call to schedule your transplant evaluation. Do not be shy to call the center to prompt their scheduling department if you have not heard back from them. Had I not done this, I would not have known that my referral never came through.

You will be scheduled for a series of extensive medical tests. These tests are typically scheduled over a two week period. The tests consist of a chest x-ray, numerous blood tests, and cardiac and pulmonary evaluations, just to name a few. The tests are intended to help the transplant center evaluate you for potential medical problems, such as heart disease, infections, bladder dysfunction, ulcer disease, obesity and transmittable diseases, like human immunodeficiency virus or HIV, hepatitis and cytomegalovirus or CMV.

You will get a chance to meet individuals on the transplant team, which is a great time for you to ask questions and obtain information about the procedure and their surgical success rate.

A social worker will also evaluate your mental and social stability. This will include discussions regarding your financial and family support needs. A financial counselor will address anticipated costs and insurance coverage, so that you will be better prepared for any out-of-pocket medical expenses and immunosuppressive drugs post-surgery.

Blood Type Compatibility

Initial tests involve a blood type screening test to determine your *blood type and tissue type*. This will help you identify who the potential living kidney donors can be. Because of the importance of blood type, be sure you have confirmation in writing from a lab before assuming what your blood type is. This is something that you can't

105

afford to get wrong when you are contemplating potential living kidney donor offers. It's not like you can change their blood type with a bottle of hair dye, or get it altered by a seamstress.

Blood type is like a genetically encoded fingerprint that requires compatibility. In direct living kidney donor transplants, the donor's blood type must be compatible to your blood type.

There are various blood types and their meaning for you as a potential kidney transplant recipient is significant when it comes to donor compatibility:

- *Blood type O*— *Recipients with blood type O can only receive a kidney from a blood type O donor. (While blood type O recipients can only receive from an O donor, blood type O donors can give to any blood type).*

- *Blood type A*—*Recipients with blood type A can only receive a kidney from a blood type A or O.*

- *Blood type B*—*Recipients with blood type B can only receive a kidney from a blood type B or O.*

- *Blood type AB*—*Recipients with blood type AB can receive a kidney from a blood type A, B, AB or O (AB is the universal recipient because they are compatible with any other blood type).*

If you have a living kidney donor who happens to be an incompatible blood type with yours, (which occurs in about 1/3 of all willing kidney living donors) then they can consider donating through a *paired exchange program.*

Paired Exchange Programs

The *paired exchange program* is a sophisticated kidney computer matching program that matches up an incompatible donor with a more suitable recipient. The incompatible living kidney donor is matched within a national database for a blood type compatible recipient — *in exchange* for a blood type compatible living kidney donor (counterpart) for you.

This paired exchange program allows incompatible blood type donors to donate a kidney to an unknown recipient, so their child, spouse, sibling, partner, loved one or friend can obtain a more suitable match in exchange for their donation.

Paired exchange programs, like The National Kidney Registry, recently celebrated their record breaking *Paired Donation Domino-Chain* involving 60 donors and recipients. As reported by the *New York Times* on February 19, 2012, this amazing *Domino Chain* of events all began with a computer algorithm and an altruist. The altruist kicked-off the chain by stepping up anonymously to donate to someone they never met.

The domino response utilizes the altruist to start a string of never-ending matches for donors and recipients. This is accomplished through very sophisticated computer software programs.

The program used by the National Kidney Registry is said to gather an astounding number of combinations — a million viable combinations — at the rate of 8,000 per second.

107

After certain groups are formed, the chain only pauses long enough to gather the next matched set of suitable donors and recipients for subsequent groups to be connected.

The heroic valor of living kidney donors entering into a paired exchange programs is felt well beyond the patient they intended to help. Through the domino effect, they end up helping those who are struggling to find a match to be exposed to a much larger pool of potential donors. This dramatically increases their recipient's chance of getting a transplant quicker and from a more suitable donor. This opportunity can minimize advanced illness, comorbidities and mortalities for those waiting.

Domino chains are not new to the transplant world. They were first performed at Johns Hopkins in 2005, and the practice of paired donation dates back to 1986 when United States Senator, Charlie Norwood (D-GA), suggested supportive legislation be passed.

Norwood, a dentist and a strong advocate for organ donation due to his own struggles with lung cancer and subsequent lung transplant went to battle to get the bill passed. Sadly, though, the cancer spread to his liver which caused his death. Yet, before passing, Norwood wrote a letter to Congress asking that the Paired Kidney Donation bill that both he and Senator Carl Levin (D-MI) introduced be sponsored by Congressman Jay Inslee. Because of that action, it did in fact become law.

Just two weeks after Norwood's death, Congressman Inslee's mother died from kidney disease, which, no doubt, gave the Congressman an urgent motivation to reduce mortality rates for all kidney patients struggling to find a compatible donor.

The Senate not only passed Senator Levin's Paired Kidney Donation bill, S.478, by unanimous consent, but one month later, the House of Representatives passed their own Paired Kidney Donation bill.

Congress renamed the final legislation in Norwood's memory, as The Charlie Norwood Living Organ Donation Act H.R. 710. It carried by a vote of 422-0. It is estimated that paired donations will one day allow for an additional 3,000 living donor renal transplants per year in America.

Paired donation follows the same initial testing protocols as followed in *direct donation*. The only difference comes down to donor matching.

Tissue Testing & Antibodies

In addition to blood type compatibility, there's a second level of matching for *tissue-typing*, called the Human Leukocyte Antigen test, or *HLA*. This is a test to determine genetic markers. Your genetic markers are located on the surface of your white blood cells. You inherit a set of three markers called *antigens* from your mother and another three from your father.

The goal is to achieve the highest number of matching antigens with your donor. While antigen matching is not a prerequisite, it is believed that a higher level of antigen matches can improve long-term outcomes.

> You inherit a set of three markers called antigens from your mother, and another three from your father.

109

There is yet another test to identify the level of *antibodies* in your immune system. Antibodies are produced to protect you by attacking foreign substances, such as bacteria and viruses. For example, your body is prompted to make antibodies to fight an infection. Your body can also develop antibodies through a pregnancy or after receiving a blood transfusion, or from a prior transplant.

Antibodies can tirelessly complicate and challenge the donor matching process. The goal here is to have low to zero antibodies, and of course, zero antibodies against your donor's *HLAs*.

If your tests reveal antibodies to your donor, then that donor would be disqualified because your body would attempt to destroy their donated kidney. When this is the case, your donor could still be considered as a potential donor for you if they are open to donating through a *paired exchange*.

Though rarely used, *plasmapheresis,* a process of stripping harmful antibodies from your blood, is another option that can be considered, both before and after transplant when there is blood incompatibility. In essence, the *plasmapheresis* process *tricks* the body into accepting the new organ which reduces the chance of rejection. The thought here is to give the body a period of time to acclimate to the new organ so it can develop a comfort zone. It's important to note however, that the process can be taxing and costly, and in some cases, the patient's spleen, which is the body's repository for antibodies, must be removed. Yet there is a drug available now that can be administered to avoid the necessity of spleen removal.

When the transplant evaluation is complete, the transplant team will meet and discuss your results with a dedicated committee. This *Selection Committee* consists of a multi-disciplinary team which includes a Transplant Surgeon, Transplant Nephrologist, Transplant Nurse Coordinator, Social Worker, Patient Financial Services Coordinator, Registered Dietician and Transplant Pharmacologist, also known as Pharm.D.

Financial Considerations

While meeting with the financial coordinator, be sure to ask questions so you'll have an idea of what to expect. They should be able to give you an idea of what your insurance will cover and what you will be responsible for by helping you better understand your benefits.

Pay particular attention to co-payments for all your medical procedures, hospital stay and prescription drugs after your transplant. Be aware of deductibles, maximum out of pocket, co-pays and annual coverage if there is a limit.

Be sure you also understand how to apply for benefits, such as ESRD Medicare benefits. You are eligible if you or your spouse have met the required work credits under the Social Security, Railroad Retirement or as a government employee. Likewise, a dependent child of a person who has met these requirements is also eligible.

With respect to transplants, the effective date is the month the individual is admitted to a Medicare certified hospital for a kidney transplant. When care is needed prior to the transplant, eligibility begins that month,

111

providing your transplant takes place within the following two months. Likewise, if your transplant was delayed for two months, eligibility would begin two months prior to the transplant. surgery.

When you have health insurance through an employer health group plan, Medicare's Coordination of Benefits, *or COB*, states that your primary insurance with your employer is primary for 30 months, and Medicare is secondary. At the end of the *COB* period, Medicare becomes the primary and the employer's group plan will be secondary for the last 6 months, if you are under the age of 65.

Immunosuppressive drug benefits will terminate at the end of 36 months, starting with the month of your transplant, if you are under the age of 65. Ask about your options for pre-planned fundraising and learn how to skillfully negotiate with insurance carriers, case managers and employers for increased benefits.

Comparatively, Medicare doesn't kick in for four months after treatment begins for in-center hemodialysis. Perhaps that's another reason to proactively be seeking a living donor well in advance of need. For more information visit:

http://www.kidney.org/professionals/cnsw/pdf/ESRD_medicare_guideli nes.pdf

Getting Listed

The multi-disciplinary *Section Committee* reviews all results from your transplant evaluation and together make a determination about whether transplant is best for you. If all goes well, you will be eligible to be placed on the transplant waiting list as a transplant recipient waiting for an eligible deceased donor.

Every person on the waitlist is registered with the United Network of Organ Sharing, UNOS, a *private nonprofit* organization, engaged under Federal Government contract for a deceased organ donor match. (Even if you think you have the perfect living donor, you want to be on the list so you get credit for your time waiting, as you never know the outcome of potential donors until you are off the operating table).

UNOS, is also a part the Organ Procurement and Transplantation Network or *OPTN*, which is a very sophisticated, centralized computer network system that links all organ procurement organizations or *OPO's*, and transplant centers to one another. *OPO's* are organizations that obtain deceased donor organs after surgical removal, and transports those organs to the designated hospital for processing and transplantation.

While *UNOS* allows multiple registrations at more than one transplant center, you may want to consider the following facts first:

a. The less time an organ is out of the donor's body before placement in the recipient's body, the better chance it has of working well. When you have a living donor, it would be best to have both surgeries performed in the same center, at the same time.

b. All transplant centers have various wait times and some move faster in some geographic areas than others. If you have the ability and financial resources to travel to other centers, then you can consider being evaluated and listed at multiple centers in different regions of the country.

c.   If you opt for multiple center registration, there is a good chance that you will be required to duplicate transplant evaluation tests. This stipulation can make multiple registrations less appealing. Travel time must also be considered, should you get "the call" and need to get to the center immediately.

d.   When considering multiple listing, be sure to coordinate with your original transplant hospital in order to manage insurance, financial and travel complexities.

e.   The waiting time that you have incurred at the center where you are currently listed can be transferred to another transplant center in another region, if you wish to change centers rather than multiple list.

f.   Deceased donor organs are offered locally, regionally and then nationally, except in cases of a perfect match, where the possibility of a successful outcome is high. You should research outcomes and waiting times at other centers you are considering before *jumping ship.*

There are many factors that go into the length of your wait for a deceased organ from the national transplant list, although the average wait does appear to be around four and a half years. Kidneys are currently allocated based primarily on how long a candidate has been waiting. Initially, the allocation system was heavily weighted based on how closely a candidate "matched" a kidney by tissue-type.

Yet now with improvements in anti-rejection medications, the need to use tissue-typing has decreased greatly. Though the debate still continues on how to modify allocation guidelines to minimize deaths for those waiting, there is equal concern for a system that allocates to promote maximum survival post-transplant as well.

The Kidney Transplantation Committee, under direction from the OPTIN Board of Directors, has been in the process of redesigning a new kidney allocation system for several years now. There have been public hearings, public forums and presentations to stakeholders. I have submitted comments and opinions over the years as a CKD patient and I encourage you to do the same when given the opportunity. Our voices must be heard.

Patients who are waitlisted at centers in high ESRD patient populations, like metropolitan areas of California and New York, can be looking at a wait of eight or more years. And, as you can imagine, waiting even a month is too long when you need a kidney today.

The biggest risk of waiting is that your illness can advance to a more serious illness— or even death. Often times as your illness advances, you lose the status that once qualified you for transplant and your name is taken off the list.

115

The Waiting Game

As previously discussed, once you have been approved by the transplant center for a kidney transplant, your name is added to the national kidney transplant waiting list. This is when the waiting game begins.

Kidneys are hard to come by, especially in a nation that cannot meet its demand. With the waitlist for all organs nearing 115,000, the daily loss of life often caused by this wait is 17 deaths a day. Sadly, the majority of these victims were waiting for a kidney.

You would think that the deaths would cause the list to dwindle. Yet this is not the case. About one hundred *new* names are added to the list every day for all transplantable organs and about 80% of them are in need of a kidney. That's one name added every 15 minutes!

The primary focus once your name is put on the deceased-donor wait list *is* to hope your name gets to the top. The twisted reality here is that while hoping for the gift of life for yourself, you also need a sufficient number of qualified and consented organ donors to die – *before* you do!

Deceased-Donor Classifications

Let's take a closer look at how the deceased organ donors are classified. Deceased donors are divided into two groups:

Group 1: Brain-dead, or *BD* donors

Group 2: Donation after Cardiac Death, *DCD donors.*

BD donors are patients who are considered dead because their brain no longer functions, even though their heart continues to pump and maintain circulation with the assist of a mechanical ventilator. Organ procurement does not begin until after it has been determined that the patient cannot breathe on their own and their wishes have been confirmed. Once the patient is taken off the ventilator to confirm BD, they are then put back on the ventilator so surgeons can start operating while organs are still being perfused.

DCD donors are patients that may still have brain function, but their heart has stopped pumping. Once their heart has stopped, there's no blood flow to the brain. This causes them to have an absence of responsiveness, heart sounds, pulse and respiratory effort. If the patient has a "do not resuscitate" order and they are an organ donor, organs can be removed as soon as the patient has been declared dead, providing the organs have not gone long without oxygen.

(Note: One deceased organ donor can save up to seven lives through organ donation — and 50 more people can be helped through tissue donation).

The miracle in *living donation,* is that the donor is still living — and quite healthy I might add. In fact, it's the only way they'd qualify.

Once you have been approved for a transplant-- and are officially listed on the National Kidney Transplant List, your approved living kidney donor completely sets you free from the waiting list by ending your dependence. At this point, both surgeries can be scheduled without further delay, providing there are no health changes.

How To Estimate The Wait

To find a list of US Transplant Centers visit: *http://www.ustransplant.org/Calculators/KidneyWaitTime.aspx.* The link also provides an instant snapshot of the approximate wait times for *deceased-donor* transplants after selecting a zip code and your preferred center. This data instantly gives perspective on the value of living kidney donation—which bypasses the wait altogether.

Wait Not: Preemptive Kidney Transplants

While living donors end the wait, you still need to find one and hope that their tests prove that they can be a candidate and suitable match for you. This process, in and of itself, can appear to be daunting to say the least. But fear not. If you are starting to follow the advice in this book before dialysis dependency—preemptive renal transplant, or *PRT*, will soon be within your reach.

Let me refresh your memory as to why preemptive renal transplant is so advantageous:

1. First, observational studies support the use of PRT as a more advantageous strategy for patients than transplantation after dialysis initiation. This is because survival and quality of life strongly support *PRT* as the optimal initial form of renal replacement therapy.

2. Dialysis dependency is often caused from the

118

wait for a deceased kidney donation. It is believed that an unclear understanding about the advantages of *PRT* among healthcare providers - and their patients, leads to delays in timely referrals which potentially squelch *PRT* possibilities.

3. According to a March 2003 article in the American Journal of Transplantation entitled: *Preemptive Renal Transplantation: Why Not?* by Mange and Weir, *PRT* optimizes a patient's ability to avoid *dialysis-associated* morbidities, such as:

   a. Hospitalizations related to dialysis access problems and infections.
   b. Cardiac disease risks related to duration of dialysis.
   c. Other health risks related to duration of dialysis.
   d. Increased T-cell reactivity related to duration of dialysis.

In addition, suspicion of a cellular phenomenon is suspected as to why PRT shows *decreased* rates of acute rejection.

You'll be pleased to know that you're paving the path for this process just by embracing the concepts discussed up to now in this book. Even better, you'll be given step-by-step instructions in *Chapter 10*, on how to attract a living donor by becoming a *Donor Magnet®*. For now, all you need to do is to share your story.

Are you surprised that I didn't ask you to ask

someone to be your donor? The good news is that you shouldn't ever have to if you follow the guidelines and tips I'm presenting in this book.

Ultimately, donors will find you!

The most effective thing you can do right now, if you haven't already done so, is to make your friends and family aware of your declining renal function. This can occur during casual conversation or at social gatherings when you are asked: "How are you?" *or* "What's new?" *(More on this in Chapter 10).*

Honoring Our Heroes

Be reminded, that even though you may feel deeply compelled to do something nice for your donor, the 1984 National Organ Transplant Act prohibits you from doing so. And although, new bills have been in play to increase donor participation by amending this Act, they have been poorly supported for fear of ethical violations.

Ethics should not be a concern if the incentive was government controlled. Likewise, using ethics to prevent the saving of lives becomes a conflict in our nation's moral responsibility.

For years our government has given its citizens tax incentives for other acts of good, like keeping the environment green and saving energy. Why should this be any different? Should the goodness of the act be diminished because someone received a reward in return? Don't we live in a society that rewards our children for good behavior? Why should it be any different for adults?

It takes a special person to donate a kidney and not everyone can do it. In fact, very few can pass all the scrupulous psychological and medical tests. Does the government really think that someone would donate a kidney for the wrong reasons just to get a tax credit? I think not.

I believe the perfect reward, which has been suggested, is lifelong medical insurance. Now there's a reward that makes sense. The donor risks their life to save another—and, although it doesn't happen often, they could even risk being denied health insurance after donation. What better way to reward the living kidney donor than to give them the security of health coverage for their selfless act? *How can that type of reward be unethical?*

It's the perfect fit and it's a win-win, because the cost to the government would be outweighed by the savings otherwise spent on dialysis, which is currently billed and paid for by Medicare.

It is estimated that CKD costs the federal government $30 billion a year, about 6% of Medicare's budget. It is also estimated that for every dialysis patient a living kidney donor untethers from machine dependency, Medicare saves $500,000 to $1 million dollars. Considering a kidney transplant surgery costs about $100,000 to $200,000, it behooves the government to consider this option for their own cost savings benefit alone. In essence, saving lives also saves money.

The argument against donor rewards appears even more outlandish when our country is suffering from an escalating budget deficit. When a promising plan to mitigate our life-threatening organ shortage comes along, one would think the government would welcome it for the cost savings alone.

Perhaps an example I recently heard might underscore the absurdity of this concern. Take salaried firefighters who risk their lives by running into burning buildings to save the lives of others. Are they any less heroic than a volunteer firefighter with the same job description? How about the patriotism of our serviceman who receive military compensation for keeping our country out of harm's way? I believe the heroic acts of living kidney donors should be viewed in the same light.

Life-Changing Wisdom Tips

1. The technology for successful kidney transplant has improved dramatically since the first live transplant was performed in 1954. Today immunosuppressive medications, blood tests and antibody testing virtually ensure a successful kidney transplant for all patients.

2. Be prepared to encourage your nephrologist to refer you for a transplant evaluation as early as possible–preferably around 25 GFR so you have the time to accommodate donor testing (more about this in later chapters).

3. Do your homework so you will be prepared to direct the referral by requesting which center you would like to be referred to.

4. Know your own blood type. Don't wait until your evaluation. Even if you think you know what it is, verify it by asking your doctor to test it again until you have confirmation in writing.

5. Understand the difference between a direct donation, where donor and recipient have compatible blood types, and a paired exchange, so that you can understand who might be or not be a suitable living donor.

6. Recognize the power of the paired exchange program and how it can help you and others.

7. Find a transplant center. Review your center's success rate and see how many patients are waiting to project your own wait time. Visit this website: *http://www.SRTR.org*

8. Compare the wait for a deceased-donor kidney, with the thought of bringing your own living kidney donor to the table. Lean into the possibility of becoming a living Kidney Donor Magnet® and start visualizing that path today. (More on this in Chapter 11.)

9. Use this life-changing wisdom to shift your fate—and prepare to live your best life!

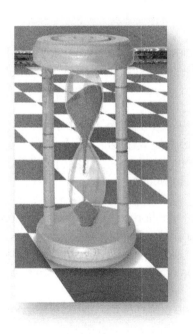

" If You Care Enough
For the Result, You Will
Almost Certainly Attain It."

– *William James*

Chapter 8: Getting Your Game Face On

Intentional Prerequisites

Now that you've arrived at this juncture in the book, there's just one prerequisite that YOU must meet, before speed-reading ahead. You must want, with all of your heart, mind and soul, to live the best life possible.

Reader Beware: It's going to take the determination of a mountain climber to scale the peaks that will soon be in front of you if you want to execute a proactive plan to *shift your fate*.

Don't be alarmed by that statement. All you need to have is desire to live your best life possible. What's your outlook right now? Are you hopeful or have you become dispirited about your situation? Either way, shake-up your thoughts by examining the following question:

> *"If You Were Given The Chance*
> *To Change Your Fate,*
> *Would You?"*

My hope is that your answer is a resounding "Yes." If you're not sure of the answer because it doesn't seem possible, then I suggest you re-read the forward by Melissa Blevins-Bein and review some of the recipient and donor stories at the end of this book.

If the answer is no, then I ask you to look deeper and ask yourself if your family doesn't deserve to experience the *best possible you*—even if you still aren't sure you want it, deserve it or can even achieve it.

If you're still on the fence about doing anything other than what you're doing right now, then allow me to rephrase the question:

"Would you embrace a cause worth fighting for,
if it could lead you to your best life possible?"

If the answer is a resounding *yes*, then put yourself on first base and get ready to develop a plan that will cause your team a winning homerun.

If the answer is no at this time, consider putting the book down for a week or so before re-examining these questions. While doing so, share some of the information you picked up with others who might benefit from these concepts. Discussions like these might be all that is needed to get you back in the game.

Spring-Board with Passionate Conviction

As you move forward in the pursuit of your best life, create a plan to <u>P</u>roactively <u>E</u>mpower <u>B</u>est <u>O</u>utcomes. Here's an exercise to help you prepare for a successful journey:

1. Start by grabbing the file with all that CKD information you've been compiling over these past months or years and give it a good look over. If you don't have a file, then look in that closet or

127

box, or wherever you've been stashing those "good to know" articles. If you don't have any of these resources to pull from, then do a search on the Internet and print out a few pages.

2. Take some time to huddle over the information for at least 20 to 30 minutes, highlighting all the key points. Yet, this time read the information as if you were reading it for the first time, even if its been your 100th time.

3. While you are putting fresh eyes to this material, cultivate a renewed interest in what you're reading. Read the copy as if you were reading into an old friend's condition—not yours. Approach the situation as Peter Falk would, as he played his role as *Lieutenant Columbo*. Scratch the side of your head and start asking what might appear to be ignorant questions on the surface, realizing all along that this is necessary work that will move your investigation forward, just like *Columbo* used to do. Framing this exercise around a friend, rather than yourself, allows you to approach the information less emotionally.

4. As you eagerly seek to learn more for your imagined friend, search for ways you might be able to help your friend. Now, imagine you found a way to help and imagine telling your friend that

you are going to help by doing everything within your power to do so.

5.   Now, ask yourself,

> *"If this was true and I did have a friend in need—and I did have the ability to help, would I?*

6.   If the answer is yes, then repeat these words out loud even if you are not sure how you will help. The point is that you want to be of service.

> *"I want to help my friend who has this condition!"*

7.   Now, repeat what you just said and say it louder and with more conviction.
     Say the following statement out loud with the same intention:

> *I'm going to find a way to help my friend!"*

8.   Say it a second and a third time, each time getting more fired up about it, as if you're playing the role of *Peter Finch* in the movie *Network*, whose most famous line was,

> *"I'm as mad as hell and I'm not going to take it any longer!"*

When you get *pumped-up good and mad,* your energy can boost pro-action.

Use this energy to transform those long held thoughts of dreadful outcomes into empowered intentions for a better tomorrow.

Is it time for you to get *pumped up good and mad* about your own situation? From what you've read thus far, I'd imagine you might already be there.

Flip It Right

Take this concept of you wanting to rescue your dear friend— and *flip it* so that the friend in need is YOU!

Now ask yourself:

> *"Am I willing to help myself as much as I would help a dear friend?"*

Hearing your own words can be extremely powerful. Knowing what you would do for someone else can be equally powerful. Simply recognize, that if you were willing to do this for someone else, then you would be able to do it for yourself. In fact, it would be foolish and even shameful, not to do it for yourself!

Still struggling? Oddly enough, a good number of people like yourself struggle with the idea of taking care of themselves, before they take care of others. Often times we are conditioned to help others, while ignoring our own self. Often times we don't realize that the gift we may be holding back from ourselves *is* a gift we're holding back from those who love us too.

Your loved ones certainly don't want your health and spirit to deteriorate. They deserve more than that from you!

Consider your spouse or significant other, children, parents, best friends and even your colleagues and employers. Don't they deserve to experience you at your best too?

If the thought of helping yourself appears to be too selfish, think again. This is not just about you. It's about you and all those around you who play a significant role in your life.

> **Your loved ones certainly don't want your health and spirit to deteriorate.**

It's time to shift away from any thoughts of self-worth, shame, denial or fear and to transcend into a new paradigm of consideration for all those concerned. Simply put—helping yourself is the right thing to do for yourself and for others.

The choice is yours. You can be *All In* so that you can embrace this new path that will lead you to your best possible life, or you can simply live your remaining years, months or days down-spiraling into what you think is a grim and pre-determined dead-end road.

Which would you choose?

Do not let your belief in your inability to find a donor or to get a transplant be relevant here. This is a conversation about taking new steps to your best life path. You can't possibly be a naysayer until you examine the steps forthcoming in the next chapter. Give them a look over before you finalize your opinions. This exercise will be well worth your time.

Taming Your Failure-Formula Tiger

Before you consider diving into the proactive steps that soon will follow, take a few moments to tame your failure-formula tiger. What is your failure-formula tiger? It's different for each person. Mine went something like this:

Panic— Fear— Surrender—Inaction

My greatest fear of course was kidney failure. My image of kidney failure was tantamount to my father's experience with kidney failure. As previously mentioned, my father was forced on dialysis in his late thirties. I witnessed him suffering catastrophic issues with his fistula and an avalanche of circumstances that followed. He then dropped into a state of depression which advanced into apathy. I believe his mental state exacerbated his illness more than his physical symptoms although his physical symptoms were causing his dispiritedness. It was a no-win situation to say the least.

If I only knew then, what I know now, things could have been so much better. If he, or I, had access to a book like this, we could have done so much more. Instead, I felt helpless. I did nothing more than watch his lifeless spirit and body deteriorate.

As I reflect back on all the inertia that overwhelmed me at that time, coupled with all my subsequent non-action when my brother was diagnosed, I feel sadness and regret. No doubt, these memories empowered my resolve to not let anyone else needlessly suffer from a lack of information.

I want all CKD patients and their friends and family to grab hold of these tools as if your life depended on it. This way you can work together to do something positive about your situation—before it's too late.

Timing is everything. Pay close attention to the opportunities that stand before you, as you may never get a second chance to look back at them again.

Be determined not to let this disease kidnap your spirit. Become a cross between *Peter Falk* from *Columbo* and *Peter Finch* from *Network*. Be inquisitive while being good and mad. Refuse to accept anything but the best route for yourself.

Believe that there *IS* something you can do—and start doing it now! You can take the first step by simply recognizing that your doctor isn't telling you everything you need to know. There's just not enough time in your appointment to do so, even if he or she tried. This is

> **Believe that there IS something you can do—and start doing it now!**

where this book comes in. Allow it to be the tour guide on this proactive exploration that you are about to take part in.

I didn't know my doctor wasn't telling me everything I needed to know, until I discovered there was more to know. It didn't hit me until I searched and studied and attended conferences to see what was out there. The new information actually released the heavy weight I was carrying around since the day I was diagnosed. This information was the power I was seeking for my entire adult life. It was truly life-saving.

This is what I hope for you.

How are you going to make the shift? Has this book caused you to think differently? Have you identified your failure formula, so that you can tame its tiger? Are you ready to release your fear and take back the wheel?

Take a moment to write out those things you think you do to self-sabotage your path and give yourself permission to let them go.

Stay The Course!

Remember, you are the CEO of your mind and body. Don't worry if you haven't quite fully adapted to that concept yet. I had to reinforce my intentions almost daily before I could get them to stick.

You cannot replace one habit, without taking on another. Let that new habit be the more proactive, inquisitive and committed you. After a while, this will all become somewhat second nature, just like wearing in a new pair of shoes. It hurts a bit at first, so you wear them just around the house to break them in. After a short while they conform to the shape of your foot quite nicely. You will soon see how your intentions will do the same.

This is not to say that the timeline to adapt to new behavior will be the same for everybody. The only thing I know for sure is that change requires daily feeding to grow strong roots. This is why it is so important to come from a state of mind that resonates with your intention. When you are "All In" you're *ready and able* to give it all you got to achieve the best outcome.

Believe me, adopting this mindset will be one of the most powerful things you'll ever do to protect your quality of your future.

Strengthening Your Power of Choice Muscle

You can strengthen your power of choice simply by becoming more informed. Having the power of choice can make all the difference in the world. By this I mean that information will reveal new concepts, and new concepts will lead you to new opportunities, which will lead you to unparalleled possibilities.

The goal is to get informed and then use that well thought-out and respected information to guide your

135

choices. Do not allow ignorance or fear of the unknown to drive choices from this point forward.

Acclimate to new behaviors in the form of a daily ritual, much like a workout routine. Simply wake up each morning and choose to be *All In*. As you say those words upon waking, commit to learning something new every day about how to avoid dialysis—or how to get off of dialysis quicker. Keep a diary or journal detailing all the reasons why you want to avoid dialysis, or stay dialysis free.

The more you learn, the more you will be able to control the little voices in your head from taking over. Simply refuse to be body-snatched by those imaginary voices that say, you don't have to do anything because you're not sick enough yet. Or the voice that says, "There's no hope, so just forget about tomorrow!" Get as good and mad as hell and say, "Enough is enough! I'm taking over now!"

Now is the time for you to take back the wheel. Navigate your journey with a refreshed outlook towards the best possible outcome. Don't let those non-alarmist perceptions trick you into believing that you have lots of time to consider your future. Optimize the time you have today, without an anxiety-driven sense of urgency.

The old adage that *"Information is power"* couldn't be more true for patients with a chronic disease. My information gathering is what caused me to reassess patient compliancy. The compliant patient only does what their doctor tells them to do, when told to do it. I'm not suggesting that you not follow what your doctor says. I am suggesting, however, that you can do more. This is about learning more on your own, so you can think for yourself while partnering with your doctor.

I am proud to be living proof that this strategy is powerful and it works! Now it is your turn. Hop into your imaginary driver's seat and release the gears from park into drive..

Stay focused on the view ahead and don't look back. Grasp your fingers tightly around the steering wheel and repeat these words out loud:

"Hello World! Meet the new me! I'm fully engaged with the intention of driving my best outcome home."

Best of all, you don't have to be in your car while doing this, although it's okay if you are. You can apply this exercise every morning before your head leaves the pillow. Just shout out your intentions for the day:

"Good Morning World!
... Just in case you're wondering,
I'm All In Today!"

Embrace this mantra as a daily ritual and before you know it things will start looking brighter. Perhaps small at first, but when you set your sights high and are willing to do the work, the most wonderful things start coming your way. Inspiration guaranteed!

137

Life-Changing Wisdom Tips

1. Be willing to embrace a cause worth fighting for; a cause that could lead you to your best life possible.

2. Be willing to help yourself as much as you would help a dear friend.

3. Your belief in your ability or inability to cure your kidney disease is not relevant. This is about staying the course for your best possible life.

4. Acclimate to new behaviors so they eventually become a daily ritual.

5. Ignore the imaginary voices telling you to wait until you get sicker. Get good and mad as hell and then refuse to accept all that ridiculous rubbish.

6. Strengthen your power of choice by using information to empower you.

7. Use this life-changing wisdom to shift your fate—and prepare to live your best life!

"The Right Thoughts
And The Right Efforts
Will Bring About The Right Results."

– James Allen

Chapter 9: Sharing Your Story

It's a Conversation, Not a Speech

If you are following the guidelines, tips and scripts I've provided in this book, then you shouldn't ever have to directly ask anyone to help you. But you do need to share your story, not in a speech but rather more like a conversation, such as you and your spouse might have at a dinner party or when you're updating the group on a recent happening, or when you're sharing a story about something your kids are going through at the time.

Through your story and through following the *Donor Magnet®* system presented here, donors will find you *(see Chapter 10)!*

The most effective thing you can do right now, if you haven't already done so, is to make your friends and family aware of your declining renal function. As previously mentioned, this can happen in casual conversation or at social gatherings when you are asked what's new *(more on this in Chapter 10)*.

These types of conversations elicit "real-life" story-telling in a natural, relaxed and genuine way. Story telling also provides you with the opportunity to discuss other aspects of why you're choosing transplant over dialysis.

Points to bring up include the difference between dialysis and transplant, the situation

> **The most effective thing you can do right now is to make your friends and family aware of your declining renal function.**

140

with the nation's organ shortage and the long wait that can be expected for a deceased donor. Be certain that you are well versed on these facts before attempting to educate others.

Don't think that sharing your story is pointless because if someone really wanted to help they would have already done so. This is foolish and self-sabotaging thinking.

The truth is that no one will ever offer to help you if they:

1. *Don't fully understand your situation.*
2. *Haven't realized they can donate a kidney while they are still living.*
3. *Aren't aware of the medical advancements in donor surgery and the low risks associated with the procedure.*
4. *Are unaware of the fact that healthy people can live a normal healthy life with just one kidney.*
5. *Are not aware of your blood type (or their own for that matter).*
6. *Are unaware that they didn't have to be blood-related.*
7. *Didn't realize there's a paired program, should they be blood-type incompatible.*

They need to learn these things about you before the thought occurs to them that they might be someone who could help.

Fortunately, friends and family often ask you how you are, so you have the perfect lead-in to tell your story as part of your answer. With that type of lead-in, you can transform a normal dialogue into telling your story. And you can turn that story-telling opportunity into a fully engaged conversation.

At any given time, depending on how the conversation is going, you can advance to more information, like what's involved in the donor's testing or the recovery timeline. But only do so if you feel the listener would be receptive.

Keep in mind that until others truly understand all the aspects to be considered, they can't begin to imagine how they could help you — or help you find someone who can.

Here are some key talking points that will help advance your dialogue:

- Describe your incurable kidney disease and the fact that you will need of a kidney transplant soon, if not already.
- Describe all the reasons why you don't want to live a life on dialysis.
- Point out the benefits of getting a kidney transplant when you need it most and the life-threatening risks associated with waiting.
- Describe your hopes and dreams of finding a living donor *before* you are tethered to a dialysis machine.
- Let them know that over 90,000 people are waiting for a kidney ahead of you.
- Describe how living kidney donors can END YOUR WAIT.
- Describe how kidneys from living donors can offer nearly twice the years in function — and can also offer superior function and outcomes,

142

when compared to deceased donated kidneys in patients who were transplanted post-dialysis.

Remember, your primary goal is to simply share your story. Stick to the facts, like when you were diagnosed, that the disease is incurable and what your concerns are about dialysis and the wait.

And before you talk to anyone, be sure to write your script and rehearse it over and over until you are comfortable with the thought of telling it to others. Doing so will help you communicate in a knowledgeable and straightforward manner—while grounding you in an information mode, rather than an asking mode.

As previously noted, you shouldn't have to ask someone to be your donor. That's way too much for anyone to ask anyone to do. It also can be overwhelming for anyone to consider when asked. If your story is not purely information based, the conversation might be construed as a donor plea, which could cause listeners to question if you have inappropriate motives, particularly if they felt pressured.

Anyone who says "Yes," under pressure, will be immediately disqualified once that fact is revealed during their donor evaluation. So, unless you want a surefire way to disqualify a potential donor, never say or do anything that would cause anyone to feel that they had to step forward on your behalf, because nobody else would.

By sticking to the facts about you and your situation, add some opinions and some heartfelt thoughts and you're on your way. If nothing else, you'll be increasing awareness and creating tremendous goodwill BUZZ for *all* those in need.

Keep your focus on the collaborative *good* you can do here, and you might be as surprised as I was, when you see what comes back your way!

Don't Ask, Tell

It was a HUGE relief for me to discover that I didn't have to ask someone to consider being my donor. No doubt, this will be a big relief for you too. If you're asking for anything, you're asking for others to help you spread the word about your story.

As soon as I understood that I didn't have to actually ask anyone to consider testing, a huge weight was lifted off my shoulders. This is when I became even more enthused about sharing my story.

> If you're asking for anything, you're asking for others to help you spread the word about your story.

While I had a purpose and I hoped to find an ideal donor, I tried to keep my focus on expanding my circle of influence through the voice of others sharing my story. At the very least, I was increasing awareness for all those in need.

Surprisingly, after the first dozen or so times I shared my story, each rendition that followed became more comfortable, more natural and more a part of me.

It was like when I first learned to ride a bicycle. The first time was a little wobbly and I needed training wheels. But with each new attempt, I got better at it until soon I was riding effortlessly all on my own. It's rather liberating to do things without a crutch. Each telling made me feel separated from my disease, just like the training wheels on my bike. I was no longer "My Disease." Sure I had it. It just didn't have me!

The more active I was in sharing my story, the more actively I received inquiries, gestures and offers. And the more inquiries, gestures and offers I received, the more determined I became to develop a system that could help others, just like you.

Getting Started

Since most healthy people don't realize that they can donate one of their kidneys (and still live a normal, healthy life), it will be up to you to get the word out. That's right. If you want to improve our anemic organ situation, your involvement is required. We all have to do our part, as there is power in the collective voice we share.

But no need to stress about this right now. You can do this—and more, by simply sharing your story and the facts surrounding it. Believe it or not, opportunities to share your story can easily flow into just about any conversation if you think about it. The most likely of which occurs quite often, just when someone asks you *how you are.*

Take advantage of this opportunity. Go beyond the typical "I'm okay how 'bout you?" response, to something like:

"Not too bad. I was just approved for a kidney transplant and I'm trying to get the word out about my need for a living donor."

145

Your story will most likely create empathetic curiosity where questions from the listener will follow. This can lead to deeper conversations, which might compel listeners to share a personal connection they have with someone who has kidney disease. Or, they may bring up other stories they've heard in the media.

Your hope is that the conversation continues, so you get an opportunity to say:

"A living kidney donor can end my wait and get me scheduled within a few months for the transplant. Yet, no one in my family qualifies. Fortunately, the donor doesn't have to be blood related, so at least the odds are in my favor to expand my options. Recently, my (friend/co-worker/spouse) offered, but they don't qualify for various medical reasons either, but I still remain hopeful."

This message gives the listener a chance to *take it all in*, so they can process their own thoughts and views surrounding the seriousness of your situation. A good and very thoughtful outcome would be that the listener says they'll include you in their thoughts and prayers. Believe me, this is a VERY good thing, so don't overlook the value in this gesture. Much good can come from this.

An even better outcome would be that they would not only include you in their thoughts and prayers, but that they would also offer to help you get the word out. This is outstanding, so once again, don't be disappointed there either. They may help you find your donor. As they ask more questions they may even consider themselves as a possibility too down the line.

Of course, the best possible outcome would be that they ask you how they can start testing to see if they would qualify to be your donor. Bingo! When this happens, your heart stops and the whole world becomes a kaleidoscope of *feel good* colors.

Be mindful that the definition of someone's offer to *help you* can vary greatly. Be sure that you understand exactly what the volunteer is saying and that they are clear on what they meant by what they just said.

For example, don't assume that they are offering to be your donor, when in fact their offer to help you may be to just help you get the word out.

> Be mindful that the definition of someone's offer to "help you" can vary greatly.

See if you can get more clarity on how they see themselves helping you. If they appear to be implying that they want to be your donor, clarify their intentions with some active listening:

"Are you saying that you'd be willing to be tested to see if you could be my donor?"

The answer to that question will eliminate assumptions and further speculation. Okay—Enough of this preamble. Let's get down to business. It's time to script your story:

Step 1: Be the Screenwriter

Pretend you're a screenwriter, scripting a movie of your life with CKD. Develop a storyboard by outlining scene objectives and goals. This will allow you to visualize the key points you want to include in your story.

Now, break out your thoughts about factual turning points in your life as a CKD patient. Don't worry about your scriptwriting skills. This is an on-going exercise. You'll be revising your drafts many times over and can perfect it then.

After you've transcribed your thoughts, read them out loud. Tweak your words if need be and then read them out loud again. Edit it as you read, if need be. Read it again out loud, and repeat the process until you feel you have something you can work with to help you write your story.

When you feel you have succinctly communicated your talking points, read it to a friend or one family member. Try it on *for size* and see how it *fits* you. Edit it as often as you like, so that it concisely communicates your situation.

The best script you can write is one that includes not only your dialogue, but also the dialogue of the party you are speaking to. This process can build your confidence and help you to be less surprised by and more prepared for unexpected listener responses.

Step 2: Rehearse it!

By rehearsing what you want to say, you'll be more likely to keep your nerves and emotions at bay. You'll also be prepared for opportunities as they arise. Rehearsing makes sharing your story in the natural course of conversation much more relaxed and natural.

While you're contemplating potential opportunities for sharing your story, try to imagine all the people and events, and all the circumstances that might allow you to share it. Visualize these venues as much as you can.

Also imagine the conversations that would accompany them, along with listener reaction scenarios. Role play each role, both listener and communicator, so that you can imagine how the listener might feel or what the listener might say, and how you would respond to their comments, questions or lack thereof.

Just as actors need to rehearse their lines, you too must become intimately familiar with what you want to say and how you will say it—preferably before the words come out of your mouth.

Your job is actually two fold. First, you want to have a story "pocket ready" so you can share it with ease, as often as you can and with as many people as possible. But there's more. You also need to tell it in a way that listeners won't get uncomfortable listening to it—or worse, feel pressured by it.

Each audience participant will process your story differently, based on their views, values and relationship with you, so be prepared for that too. They might also share their thoughts on organ donation, or even religion for that matter. Oftentimes there is a false perception that there are religious restrictions to organ and tissue donation. The fact is that nearly all religious groups support organ and tissue donation and transplantation, as long as it doesn't impede the life or hasten the death of the donor.

149

Most likely, you'll get a chance to be exposed to a variety of responses. No doubt, you'll meet up with *Opinionated Oscar* who recites political or religious beliefs about organ donation; *Empathetic Edgar* who offers to help even though he's not clear what that would mean; *Awkward Alice* who's not sure what to say, so she says nothing at all; *Interested Isaac*, who wants to learn more; and bighearted *Eager Ellie*, who sincerely wants to do something right now—no matter what it takes.

Don't be put off by those, who at the first hearing of your story, don't know how to respond, or don't offer to help you. Give them time to process.

Because this is a delicate subject, you must be prepared to tell your story and react as if you were on the side of the listener. People need time to process what they've just heard. Everyone has a place in this world. Living kidney donation isn't for everyone.

> **Don't be put off by those, who at the first hearing of your story, don't know how to respond.**

When you are writing your script, keep the above-mentioned characters in mind and use your natural style of speaking, so that when you're sharing your story it clearly comes from the heart. You don't want it to sound memorized, as if you're reading off a teleprompter.

There's no need to actually memorize your script, word for word. In fact, you're advised not to do that, for that only makes you sound too rehearsed. Simply use your script as a guide to keep you on point and keep your emotions at bay.

Keep in mind that your script is not just about telling your story. It's also about providing your listeners with the facts. Have the facts and be as up-to-date as possible. Check the latest accounting of the number of people waiting on the list ahead of you on *UNOS's OPTN* site: *http://optn.transplant.hrsa.gov/data/*

Search online for articles about our nation's life-threatening organ shortage, dialysis mortality rates, the increasing prevalence of living kidney donors and the unmatched value of preemptive kidney transplantation.

Step 3: Practice Makes Perfect

Rehearse in front of the mirror for starters. Watch your body language and pitch to avoid coming across too emotional or pushy, or worse— too needy! Rehearsing in front of the mirror can give you instant feedback. It's a terrific tool for refining your storytelling skills.

Then, after you feel comfortable with your mirror rehearsals, escalate to a telephone solicitor, the grocery clerk or the bag guy or gal. Think that's out of place? Think again. No one ever talks to them. Start by asking them how their day is going! What better way to use these opportunities then to be nice and practice your assignment.

Ask your husband or wife or even a neighbor, or a good friend to role play with you. If nothing else, they'll become more aware of your story so that they share it to.

The more you tell it, the more opportunities to increase your circle of influence. It's like a nuclear chain reaction. Each person that tells your story is inspiriting others to tell your story. This chain reaction expands the number of people who can create potential opportunities.

Step 4: Commit Once a Day

Regardless of how you plan to deliver your message, push yourself to be like *Nike®* and "just do it" —at least once a day.

Even when you get cold feet, push yourself to do it on behalf of *all* those in need. Make this about something bigger than yourself and the process becomes far more meaningful.

Make it your sense of duty. That's what I did and it worked for me. It will work for you too.

Step 5: Squelch Negative Thoughts

Don't get hung up on negative thoughts like, "Would people think I'm worthy?" or "Why should someone want to help me?" You are worthy. And believe it or not, most people want to help others—perhaps not in the ultimate way of being a living kidney donor, but in some small way, most people will want to do something to help you.

But also remember that this isn't just about you. This is about all those who stand beside you and behind you. Recognize that things will never change for the good— or ourselves for that matter, unless we change our view of the world and the role we play in it.

Shout out from the mountaintops to increase awareness about our nation's organ shortage and about all the innocent casualties it causes. Help me get living kidney donation at the top of the reader board for volunteerism, as one of life's greatest lifetime achievements. Collectively, we can make a difference, but I need your help.

Step 6: Please Do Tell!

Start sharing your story as often as you can and with as many people as possible. You decide what you want to say and how much detail you want to mention initially. You decide the best time to seize the moment of conversation.

No matter how awkward or nervous you might be about the thought of sharing your story at first, practice will make it easier. At first, it might feel as awkward as introducing yourself to an important person or group.

Initially, it's a bit nerve racking, but once you get through that initial anxiety, you'll feel back at home with yourself again.

Working from a script will be far more effective than just sharing your story with others "off the cuff." The goal here is to ensure key points are prioritized and communicated succinctly, before launching into conversation with others. This builds a comfort zone for both storyteller and listener.

Building a comfort zone in telling your story will also give your story wings. And, remember, don't just focus on you.

Paint with a broader brush by speaking on behalf of *all* those in need. When you do, the wings of your story take flight.

Step 7: Other Important Considerations

Living kidney donation is indeed catching on, yet it is still somewhat novel for most. That said, you might create some additional sound bites in your story for those times when you feel that your listener would be

153

comfortable engaging in a more philosophical discussion.

Here are some examples:

- Share headline stories featuring living kidney donors. Underscore how this concept of organ donation is much broader than donation after death.

- Share this link to a video on living kidney donation: *See new living kidney donation education video* : http://www.cpmc.org/advanced/kidney/LivingDonation/

- Share facts about deceased organ donation numbers and make it known that to be an organ donor doesn't necessarily make it so. A donor's wishes must be documented, and then they must be medically qualified to be considered at the time of death.

- Encourage open discussions on a new organ donation system much like those in several European countries. For example, in the U. S. we have what is called: **Assumed Declination**. If there is no evidence of *expressed consent* from the deceased donor, then it is assumed that the patient is *not* an organ donor—and viable organs cannot be used to save lives.

But some countries outside the U.S., follow the **Presumed Consent** law. This means, that if there is no evidence of *expressed declination* from the deceased, they are presumed to be a donor if they qualify. This policy, along with living kidney donation, has the potential to shore up organ shortages and eliminate the illegal temptation surrounding dangerous black market sales.

In presumed consent, individuals are forced to document that they are opposed to organ donation. Doing so requires action on their part. To be a donor under this system requires no action be taken. This generally results in a great number of donors.

Unfortunately, in the U.S., the majority of well-intentioned folks never get around to recording their intentions — even on the back of their driver's license. Procrastination of this kind can prevent potential donors from saving the lives of up to 8 people upon their passing.

- Another topic might include your position on supporting *zero financial impact* for living donors, up to and including lost wages for time off work and home care assistance during recovery.

Currently, under the National Organ Transplant Act, 42,U.S.C. 274e (2002) (NOTA), enacted in 1984 it is a federal crime to "knowingly acquire, receive or otherwise transfer any human organ for valuable consideration for use in human transplantation if the transfer affects interstate commerce (transfer of goods or money)." The maximum fine for this is $50,000 or a five-year imprisonment term, or both.

Fortunately, the fine print in the definition of valuable consideration states the following is *excluded* from that intent: *"reasonable payments associated with removal, transportation, implantation, processing, preservation, quality control and storage of a human organ* [which would be paid to the procurement and transplant team], *or the expenses of travel, housing and lost wages incurred by the donor of a human organ in connection with the donation of the organ."*

Yet, there is so much fear surrounding the violation of the transfer of money, that this exclusion has a proclivity to be interpreted as *all inclusive*, rather than the exception to the rule. On the state side, there is a law that also prohibits organ sales based on the Uniform Anatomical Gift Act, 8A U.L. A. 15 (1983) (UGA), which was passed by the National Conference of Commissioners on Uniform State Laws in 1968 and adopted by the District of Colombia and all fifty states (with minor variations) in 1973.

The National Kidney Foundation is a strong supporter of policies to provide donor leave and reimbursement for direct expenses related to living donation. A summary of these policies follow.

Federal Legislation

Donor Leave Laws: Employees of the federal government receive 30 days paid leave for organ donation and 7 days for bone marrow donation. The leave is over and above the employee's sick and annual leave. (HR457/Public Law 106-56).

Tax Credit *(Pending legislation)*: Legislation has been introduced that would provide a federal tax credit of up to $10,000 for unreimbursed expenses, including lost wages, for living donors of kidney, liver, lung, pancreas, intestine or bone marrow.

State Legislation

Donor Leave Laws: Modeled after federal law (for federal employees), many states have begun to offer state employees up to 30 days leave (paid or unpaid) for serving as a living organ donor. This leave is considered separate from any annual or sick leave already accrued by an employee. Eight states *(Arkansas, Connecticut, Illinois, Louisiana, Maine, Minnesota, Nebraska and Oregon)* allow a leave of absence for private sector employees, but in many cases, it only applies to marrow (not organ) donors. Usually, the period of leave is 30 days for organ donors or 7 days for bone marrow donors.

Tax Deductions or Credits*: Many states have also enacted tax deductions or credits to living donors. Wisconsin and Georgia allow living organ donors to deduct up to $10,000 in expenses from state income tax. Other states, where such legislation is pending include Illinois, Massachusetts, New Jersey, New York and Pennsylvania. (For more information see the *Resource Section* for "Waiting for a Transplant" through the National Kidney Foundation.)

*Due to evolving legislation and potential changes in the law, the accuracy of the aforementioned information could be outdated. It is paramount that your donor(s) confirm their specific state laws on living donor tax credits to ensure they have an accurate understanding of the law and its restrictions.

157

Information related to these topics can be found at:
http://www.kidney.org/transplantation/livingdonors/pdf/LDTaxDed_Leave.pdf;
http://www.kidney.org/atoz/pdf/waitingforatx.pdf

The Ad Hoc Living Donor Subcommittee of the United Network of Organ Sharing, (*UNOS*), has proposed that employers continue the compensation for employee wages otherwise lost during the medical leave for up to 30 days following hospitalization for employees who are living organ donors.

Altruism is Not Enough

Altruism is associated with words like: selfless, self-sacrifice, humanitarianism and philanthropy. Dr. Sally Satel is a published author, practicing psychiatrist and lecturer at the Yale University School of Medicine as well as a Resident Scholar of the American Enterprise Institute *AEI*. She also examines mental health policy and political trends in medicine. She explains it a bit differently when it comes to living kidney donation. She says:

> *"Altruism is a beautiful virtue but relying on it as the sole motivation for giving an organ ensures we will never have enough of them. The gift of life is priceless—people who give it should receive some material reward for their generosity. Though altruism often moves relatives and strangers to donate, strangers usually need a stronger incentive, if they are to relinquish an organ. Compensation, in some form, for organ donation, could motivate thousands of new donors to come forward—but the 1984 National Organ Transplant Act (NOTA) made it a felony to provide any material reward."*

In her book, *When Altruism Isn't Enough (AEI Press, October 2008)*, Dr. Satel argues that compensating people who donate an organ to a desperate stranger—an extraordinary act of life-saving value—will motivate others to do the same.

Dr. Satel believes the reward could potentially increase the national supply of kidneys and reduce needless death and suffering. When you think about it, there's a reward for finding a lost child for providing information to help the investigators find the child and save a life— even though it's the right thing to do anyway. So why not in organ donation?

A reward system simply puts more value on the efforts of those who could help find the person who could save a life. In organ donation the organ donor is the person saving the life. It should be no different than other cases where rewards are offered. If anything, giving up one's kidney for the sake of a stranger's life should be even more deserving of reward.

Does a paid fireman hold any less significance than the volunteer fireman who ran into the twin towers to save a life? Why should living organ donors be classified any differently if they were to be rewarded for their heroic efforts?

Dr. Satel calls on government-regulated entities to offer appropriate incentives (such as health insurance, tax credits, tuition vouchers or a contribution to a tax free retirement account) to reward individuals willing to donate a kidney to a stranger. Dr. Satel believes that because the compensation would be provided by a third party—every patient in need, regardless of income—would benefit.

Dr. Satel also believes that an incentive-based program to increase the supply of transplantable organs would also suppress unauthorized markets overseas. Such a program should not be discouraged by the government, as dollars spent basically equal dollars saved. For example, a tax benefit reward to a living kidney donor, which on the surface appears to be an expense to the government, would essentially equate into saving hundreds of thousands of dollars, which would otherwise be spent on dialysis—a necessity to keep the patient alive while waiting for a deceased donor's kidney for a transplant.

Senator Arlen Spector understood these benefits and introduced the Organ Donation Clarification & Anti Trafficking Act, *ODCAT*, of 2008. The aim was to uphold historic bans on commercial private sales of organs, while permitting states to set up a program for government compensation to organ donors. While supporters of the bill recognized the power of this life saving bill, it never became law.

Perhaps this was due in part to the concerns voiced from those who feared the poor would donate for the wrong reasons. How long must we allow unsubstantiated fears of this nature to stand in the way of preventing life-saving opportunities for the more than 4000 kidney patients who die each year while waiting?

We cannot simply stand by without letting our voices be heard. Both you and I can become human megaphones, by letting the world know that something must be done—and it must be done now. Embrace this urgent call to action for all those in need, before you find yourself on the list in imminent danger alongside them.

Life-Changing Wisdom Tips

1. Sharing your story is a conversation, not a speech—and not a plea for someone to help you. Make your friends and family aware of your declining renal function.

2. You don't have to ask someone to be your donor, but you do need to share your story and educate others about the life-threatening shortage.

3. Script your story and then rehearse it over and over again. Be sure to include educational highlights about dialysis risks and the length of the national wait for a deceased organ as well as providing heartwarming stories about living kidney donors.

4. Be certain that you fully understand the information you're sharing before you attempt to educate others.

5. While telling your story be certain to present it so listeners don't get uncomfortable— or worse, feel pressured to help you.

6. No one will offer to help you if they don't fully understand your situation or the details surrounding your circumstances. Of equal importance, they need to understand what's involved in the donor surgery and details about the recovery. (See Chapter 12.)

7. Don't be put off by those, who at the first hearing of your story, don't know how to respond. Because this is a delicate subject, be mindful of how you'd react if you were in their shoes.

8. Don't just focus on you. Paint with a broader brush by speaking on behalf of *all* those in need. Educate. Increase awareness. Give your story wings.

9. See how you can include additional information in your story as you get to repeated interactions with the same people. Invite intellectual dialogues on Assumed Consent, government issued rewards for living donors and your thoughts on how our nation can prevent unnecessary deaths.

10. Use this life-changing wisdom to shift your fate—and prepare to live your best life!

"Until Input *(thought)*
Is Linked To A Goal *(purpose)*
There Can Be No
Intelligent Accomplishment."

– Paul G. Thomas

Chapter 10: Ten Steps To Becoming A Donor Magnet®

Step 1: Seek First To Understand

If your goal is to receive a kidney transplant from a living donor so you can bypass dialysis, then seek first to understand both sides of the equation. Imagine for a moment, the character one must possess to answer such a heroic life-saving call on your behalf. Imagine what you'll feel like when offers are actually presented.

Process your feelings well before attempting to make this dream a reality. It is equally important for you to fully understand what the living kidney donor would have to go through for testing, in both surgery and throughout recovery. Have both a sense of understanding and compassion for all aspects of this process.

The more knowledgeable you become, the more successful you will be in educating others.

Remember, your goal is to enlighten, educate and inform. This focus is the best path toward emotionally intelligent conversations with potential "buzz" spreaders and donors. Create interest and

> Remember, your goal is to enlighten, educate and inform.

curiosity when sharing your story in order to invite a two way conversation that is both relaxed and meaningful.

Be mindful that you will be exposed to some individuals who get so excited about helping you that they'll jump a bit too fast. When you hear "I can do that!" before someone fully understands what's involved, you could be in for a rude awaking. For it has been said that those who jump too quickly to raise their hands don't completely understand the scope of what they just volunteered to do.

That is where the newly empowered and more knowledgeable YOU comes into play. Assume that all potential donors do not understand the scope of what they are contemplating. This awareness will remind you to always attempt to enlighten others. You can paint information in broad strokes, while encouraging them to do some research on their own. They can also talk to other living kidney donors who have *been there* before them.

> Assume that all potential donors do not understand the scope of what they are contemplating.

You can also direct them to informative website links, such as: www.kidneykinships.org/The_Donor_Process.html Also, provide them your transplant center's donor desk hotline and other resources like a copy of this book's *Chapter 11: I Think I Found A Donor. Now What?*

Your job is to merely point them in the right direction for information. Your goal is to get them linked to unbiased information sources in order to avoid the appearance of a conflict of interest.

Both parties will feel more comfortable about this information gathering process.

Step 2: Enlist Donor Advocates

Let's face it, it's hard to share your story all by yourself. It takes a village to get your message out in the world. Building a support network of friends and family will advance your process exponentially. The key here is there is more power in numbers.

165

Having others share your story (third party) is often more effective than sharing your story in first person. The indirect approach reduces the likeliness of overwhelming listeners, which can trigger them to feel pressured or say something just to make you feel better.

When selecting donor advocates, consider individuals who have compassion, emotional intelligence and a willingness to learn. Be sure to invite your team members to learn along with you. This is the best way to ensure that they will share your story and its surrounding facts with accuracy.

It's imperative that both you and your teammates are equally familiar with the donor process facts, as described in *Chapter 11*, so that they are aware of all the testing, surgical and recovery aspects involved for potential living donors. This is the only way to ensure accuracy when painting an overview of what's involved.

As your team members become fully enlightened about your story and the surrounding facts involved, ask them to start sharing your story and encouraging others to join them as **Donor Recruitment Magnets®**.

Donor Recruitment Magnets® are individuals who are actively helping you share your story by spreading the word about your need for a living kidney donor.

Remember, you need to create *buzz*. The more voices out there, the more listeners you'll reach. The more listeners you reach, the stronger your circle of influence. The stronger your circle of influence, the greater the chance for attracting those who resonate with this calling.

Step 3: Mentors & Coaches

Working with a mentor or coach can make all the difference in the world. I never realized this until I tapped into a mentor myself. Actually, I spoke to a couple of mentors, but neither one of us knew I was being mentored. I simply sought out people who I admired and who achieved what I was hoping to achieve, and I tapped into their wisdom.

I was referred to my most valuable mentor before I even knew I was looking for one. And I never realized how rich that relationship would become. Jill was a kind woman with a big heart, who generously gave of her time to help me understand my options. While I was referred to her because I was told she

> **Working with a mentor or coach can make all the difference in the world.**

was a very astute transplant recipient, I had no idea just how powerful her knowledge base was or how her wisdom would play out in my life. She literally guided me through each fork in the road, which enabled me to believe it was possible to change my fate.

Today, I am proud to call Jill both my friend and mentor. Seeking advice from Jill, instead of going it alone (*if I may put my own spin on a quote from Mark Twain*), was like the difference between lightning—and a lightning bug! I discovered more from Jill than I would have ever discovered on my own, no matter how many books I read or hours I surfed the internet.

So what is my message to you? Don't hesitate to find a mentor or coach to help you do the same. Simply ask someone you admire to mentor you. If they already offer that type of professional service, then hire them to be your patient coach.

If you don't know where to seek such enlightened individuals, you can contact the National Kidney Foundation's *(NKF's)* Peers Program or our firm, The PRO*active* Path, to inquire about our mentoring and coaching services. (For more information on *NKF's PEERS Mentor Program* or *The PROactive Path's coaching services*, see the *Resource Section* at the end of this book).

Before contacting a mentor or coach, get a feel for their philosophy and background so you can ensure you're seeking the *right fit*. Have an idea of your schedule and be prepared to ask for times that work for you. You will get the most out of your call if your sessions are scheduled in advance.

This is not the type of conversation to have by catching someone on the fly. The meeting must be preplanned and you'll need to be prepared. Begin the dialogue by thanking your mentor or coach for taking the time to speak to you. Your expression of gratitude from the *get-go* can speak volumes.

Let them know that you've put some thought into the call and that you've been assessing your CKD path, and that you now see the need for some help from someone who has already walked in their shoes.

Let them know that you feel a connection to their philosophy and that you believe in what they stand for. *(Of course you'll need to know what that is before stating this).*

If you feel a connection to their message, ask them if they would be willing to talk with you on a regular basis, and what the fee would be, if there is one.

If your mentor is fully committed at this time, don't give up. Ask them who they might recommend, of if they wouldn't mind if you check back with them periodically to see if their schedule opens up. If they already provide coaching services for a fee, let them know that you are willing to be a paying client, if you want to be able to fall into their pre-blocked *"new client"* time.

Step 4: Your Outreach Email List

It's time to plan who you want to *e*Blast your story to virtually. Even if you think that sending an email blast is premature at this time, create the list anyway and consider a mini educational awareness piece, by sharing facts on the nation's life-threatening organ shortage.

Add a heart-felt living donor story that hit the news recently, like the nurse who donated one of her kidneys to a patient in renal failure, or the taxi driver who offered to donate one of his kidneys to a women he drove to dialysis 3 times a week.

Be sure to splash a few tidbits about your diagnosis into these stories in order to personalize the message. The timing of your email will give potential recruiters ample time to help you get the word out and ample time to contemplate how they can help you.

As you get closer to the low 30s or high 20s of GFR, you can follow up with another email updating your audience about your urgent need.

For those already in Stage 4, turn up the volume by putting more emphasis on your diagnosis, your need for a kidney—and your resolve to avoid a debilitating life on dialysis.

<u>Here are some tips to help you create your list:</u>

- **Create a digital list to stay organized.** Your list should include everyone you know. Enter their names and contact information on the *Outreach List Form* found in this book's *Forms, Charts & Scripts Section*. Save the list in a file so you can use it for email execution and tracking.

- **Don't limit the list.** The list should include all individuals you know who you think might potentially help you network your story. Don't limit the list to family members and close friends.

- **Be sure to include** work associates, colleagues, and individuals you know through professional organizations, as well as those you know through church or synagogue associations.

- **Don't prejudge** anyone on how compassionate you think they are, or how busy they are. Just make the list. As many kidney transplant recipients have attested, myself included, some of the most incredible acts of human kindness have come from those we least expected.

- **Track the dates.** Be sure to track what you sent out and when, so your follow-up will be tight and seamless. As your function declines it will more challenging to remember what went out and who got what. Be sure to document your actions so you can follow-up accordingly.

Step 5: e-Blasts

After you've created your list, transform your scripted story, which by now, you should have created with your assignment from the previous chapter into written communication. If you haven't created your script yet, you'll need to go back and review the suggestions on how to script your story from *Chapter 9* first.

After you have your script in hand, transform the verbal telling of your story into a written communication. You can do this by including facts surrounding your diagnosis, the turning points, your need for a kidney transplant and your message of hope. End the communication by inviting readers to help increase awareness and be sure to invite them to contact you if they have interest in learning more.

Be sure your email blast is more of an information piece so readers won't feel pressured. Be mindful of how you'd respond if you were on the other side of this exchange. Select key individuals on your donor recruitment team to send out the *e-Blast* for you. Your teammates are often better suited to communicate your story, because they are sharing it from the point of view of a person who cares. This also removes the unthinkable task of soliciting a personal plea for help.

My husband wrote and sent my first *e-Blast* and we received some awesome feedback. We found it far easier for him to describe his view of my situation, as a caring husband who didn't want to see me suffer. He couldn't be my donor so he became one of my biggest champions, helping me find someone who could.

171

His communication style was heartfelt and reader-friendly. It gave readers a "safe zone" for communication. No one wants to disappoint you, so this third party way of communication can open communication dialogues and level the playing field for both sender and receiver.

Check out the sample template of a 3rd Party eBlast in the *Forms, Charts & Scripts* section of this book to get an idea of what the message might sound like. Note that the sample is a bit long, but I wanted to include several ideas for you to pick and choose from. Yours should be more succinct and factual, with several heartfelt layers of *feel good*. Too much information will overwhelm readers or even dissuade the reading of the piece altogether. Less is more.

Be sure that the focus of the *e-Blast* isn't just about YOU. Paint with a broader brush by speaking on behalf of *all* those in need. Underscore the sender's emotional intelligence and use expressions that fit their natural speaking voice.

Include your goals as a means to educate. Don't be shy in telling your sender what those are, so they can be communicated. Also, be sure to include important donor facts, like: (1) healthy individuals can live a full, vibrant life with just one kidney, (2) all medical expenses are covered by [insert recipient's here] medical insurance, and (3) how living kidney donors end the life-threatening wait, and (4) how living kidney donors earn a special status for themselves after donation, should they ever experience the unlikely event of needing a kidney themselves someday. This status essentially escalates them toward the front of the line to honor their selfless act of human kindness.

If you happen to have superior writing skills, ghostwrite the body of the message and then let your sender tweak it to their style. In either case, be sure to put your eyes on the document before it goes out in order to ensure the information accurately communicates your story and is typo-free.

And, last but not least, don't forget to encourage email *forwards*, so those receiving it can further increase your outreach, by forwarding it on to others.

Now, it's time to send it. Combine your *Outreach List* with additional addresses from your approved sender's *Outreach List* so that you'll be able to target a collaborative audience.

Do not overlook proper email etiquette by disclosing the addresses of the parties to whom you are emailing. Keep that information confidential. To do this, either set up an undisclosed list, or blind copy the group in the "BCC" area. Be mindful that no one wants their email address going around in group messages for both privacy reasons as well as to avoid annoying *"reply to all"* responses. It is essential to apply common courtesy here.

Be certain to document which parties were included in your first mailing. That way you will know who you sent this first communication to and when.

Before sending the eBlast, insert your story into the body of the email, re-read and proof it a couple more times. Look for proper alignment, wording and correct phrasing of sentences.

Be sure it is saying what you and your sender intend it to say, and in the way you want it communicated. Have all your buddies that you enlisted in Step 2 also review the *e*Blast for each of these items.

The more "eyes" you can put on the *e*Blast before sending it, the more you can be sure that the copy is correct and that the message is clear.

Step 6: Social Media

With today's information highway, there's no shortage of opportunity through social media communication. Vehicles such as Facebook, Twitter, LinkedIn and Google Plus have expanded the reach and power of one's voice. You can also build a dedicated website on sites like *CaringBridge.com,* or create a Blog to get your story out. Once you have a website or blog you can link those pages to your social media outlets.

But I do have one word of caution relative to the use of social media. That is, a lot of transplant centers do have issues with using social media for donor recruitment. While some don't, there are a good number that do. So, before you do a lot of work in this area, check with your intended transplant center to see what their protocols are for living donor social media connections.

If your center approves social media but you are not internet savvy, consider looking into a freelance assistant to help you.

> Be sure to check with your transplant center to see what their protocols are for living donor social media connections.

There are internet sites that can make the process of finding a contractor quite easy. The one I tend to use is Odesk.com. Here you can find copy editors, and social media experts who can expand your exposure.

You'll be able to preview specific contractors within a specific area of expertise, view their experience and portfolio information and evaluate their fee structure before hiring. You can invite individuals to your job, or you can simply post a job for public viewing and wait for proposals to come in.

Using outsourced services will free you up to concentrate on learning more and doing more for your personal campaign. You can end procrastination tendencies when you lack the time or skill to do certain things.

Whether you engage in social media on your own, work with your buddies or hire out, I have another word of caution here. Social media tends to hold a higher degree of disappointment. In other words, while the virtual donor might express that they want to help you and that they're *all in* for testing, it's not uncommon to get all your hopes up and then to never hear from them again.

Be it distractions going on in their own lives or dissuasion from family or friends, these situations can happen so it is best to prepared for them. More often than not, social media donors tend to drop out after discovering they held unrealistic expectations. And while these scenarios seem to be more prevalent in virtual relationships, it can also happen with individuals you've known for years.

Step 7: Media Exposure

This concept can be quite effective. Contact local media (i.e., newspapers and TV stations) and ask if they

175

would like a personal, local story to attach to newsworthy statistics about chronic kidney disease.

Maximize your efforts by helping the media understand how your story can impact their readers, viewers or listeners. Provide them with a *hook*, by highlighting key facts surrounding the nation's organ shortage and the lives lost daily. Better yet, be more specific and provide them data from your own state by capturing information specific to your area from *UNOS's OPTN* database link: http://optn.transplant.hrsa.gov/data/

Be sure to personalize the message by including your story, but only if you can be succinct and heartfelt at the same time. Then, tie a bow around your proposal by underscoring how the circumstances of your story and the benefit of what will come if you were to receive a kidney transplant can position this story front and center.

You can also look for events in your area that have to do with kidney awareness, such as fundraising walks or free screenings. Then you can contact the media and ask if they would like a personal and local story to attach to the event. As the Chapter Coordinator for the PKD Foundation in Phoenix, I was able to share my story on *CBS, KPHO Channel 5* in an effort to help promote our annual signature fundraising event, the *Walk For PKD*.

This was my first opportunity to share my story with the public—and fortuitously it was not my last. This story created wonderful buzz about our walk, yet it didn't create half as much interest as it did about another story the station ran shortly thereafter.

That story involved a live interview with a remarkable woman who offered to be my donor *sight unseen!* It all started with a vitamin store sales clerk named Pam, who stepped up to be my hero. Pam had befriended my mother, a customer who shopped in her store often as a proponent of natural supplements. Their interactions started with the need for Pam to help my mom, who had macular degeneration, read the labels and to give her advice. Pam was so helpful and sharp—and FUN, that they naturally gravitated to developing an in-store friendship.

Yet, on one particular visit, which shall go down in history for me, my mom had an opportunity to share my story. Since Pam hadn't seen my mother in some time, she asked where she had been hiding. The answer to that question led my mother to describe her trip to California for my brother's kidney transplant surgery. The story, from what I was told, was somewhat bittersweet. While my mom expressed joy and relief about my brother's success, she coupled it with her concern about me. This was at a time that I was getting close to needing a kidney transplant.

Not realizing that my brother would need a second transplant, my mom intended to donate one of her kidneys to me. Yet, due to her age, she was told she could not. Neither one of us ever contemplated that her age might prevent this—or that our blood types could be incompatible, which turned out to be surprisingly true.

While Pam listened to my mother's accounting of her sorrow and empathized with her pain, she jumped at the chance to help without hesitation. She said, "I'll donate a kidney to your daughter!" And that's how the story started—and almost ended, had it not been for the

Selection Committee's disqualification, which prevented her from being my direct donor.

When Pam made her mind up to do something, nothing got in her way, not even donating a kidney when the committee discouraged her from doing so. The fact is that she made up her mind to be a living kidney donor and come hell or high water, she was donating, or at least she prayed for that to be the case.

While Pam was put on hold as a potential back-up donor for me, she patiently waited for almost a year to be sure I was taken care of. As a few more potential donors stepped forward to be tested on my behalf, one by one they were all disqualified. But then, in 2010, my ideal donor revealed herself to me and subsequently passed all her tests with flying colors. This amazing blessing progressed from approved donor to surgery date in the blink of an eye.

That allowed me to encourage Pam to meet another potential recipient who I knew was in desperate need, and as it turned out, they were a better match. In 2011, Pam donated her kidney to Joyce. Because of Pam's willingness to *wait it out* and be tested yet again for another potential recipient, she was able to save Joyce from dialysis, while giving me a sense of security throughout my donor search.

And it gets even better. Pam's sister, Glenda, was so moved by Pam's desire to donate a kidney to me, that she ended up anonymously donating one of hers to a stranger the year prior to Pam's donation to Joyce. In between all of this wonderment, I received my kidney from the amazing Ms. Melissa. *(More to come on this from MAK's Blessing in Chapter 11.)*

Though Pam didn't end up being my direct donor, she gave me and so many others a gift more precious than gold or diamonds. She helped increase awareness, and she now serves as a role model for others. She will always be known to me as Angel Pam, a very fitting nickname that I gave her the day we met on March 29, 2009.

Of course, the point of these stories, in addition to all the feel-good here, is that you can get your own media exposure if you try. It's not going to happen if you just sit around and wait for it to happen. You have to be proactive and you must be *All* In! When you're determined to make a difference for yourself and others, interviews will find you, just as they did me.

Pam and I were interviewed a second time after she won the *"Pay it Forward"* award which she so duly deserved. But that didn't happen on its own either. I was a treasure hunter; I sought out opportunities. Channel 5 was running a *Pay it Forward* contest, and I submitted Pam's story. I thought, who could compete with the kindness of a clerk in a vitamin store who tried to save the life of a daughter of one of her customers?

The airing of this story caused another very special local woman to reach out and contact me to see if she could be tested on my behalf. She was so kind and thoughtful, and willing to wait weeks to be tested. She too was told that she was not an ideal candidate, yet insisted on getting a letter from her doctor to be retested.

Unfortunately, she didn't pass the retesting either, but she gave me so much hope during that time and I was deeply moved by her desire to save me from a life on dialysis. The flip side of that TV airing causes me to give you a word of caution, however, on another scenario I experienced. I was contacted by another woman who worked for a reputable state agency, after she learned about Pam not being able to donate to me. She accessed the *"Pay it Forward"* story off the TV station's web linked achieves.

It was all so surreal at first. I received an email followed by several phone calls and a friendship, so I thought, was developing. After over 8 weeks of hopeful emails, texts and promising telephone conversations, the communication ceased, and I never heard from her again. Later I discovered that she never showed up for her testing appointments either. I share this story with you, so that you don't put all your eggs in one basket. Feeling secure with one donor can be dangerously misleading and disheartening.

Step 8: Message Boards

Many places of worship and other organizations have both digital and physical reader boards that allow people to post messages. Take advantage of these free vehicles to get the word out about your need for a kidney donor.

SEEKING HEROIC VOLUNTEERS

Have you wondered what it would be like to save someone's life— or transform someone's life? Being an organ donor is an amazing thing to offer at the end of your life—and donating a piece of yourself while you are still living can be even more amazing! A member of this congregation could use your help, If you're in good health and hold interest in becoming a living kidney donor or donor advocate, please contact the member's Path Leader, Grace 555-345-6789, or email: *grace@thisisanexampleonly.com*

Step 9: Events & Opportunities

Another tremendous outreach option could be realized through fundraising events. You can host an event to increase awareness and raise money for CKD research *or* support kidney patient organizations like the American Association of Kidney Patients *or* the National Kidney Foundation, who depend on funds to provide patient aid and assistance.

If there is a foundation or support group for your specific kidney disease, you can direct your donations to fund research for your specific disease.

Fundraising events have the potential to increase awareness. They can increase awareness about your disease, your story, your need for a kidney and the nation's organ shortage. All you need is to have someone emcee the event with opening and closing comments about the event's purpose.

Don't try to *go it alone* if you are not well versed in event planning. It would be best to outsource the event to an expert in this area to make sure your event is properly planned, managed and advertised. Such experts can ensure that you get the right media exposure too.

If there is an opportunity to volunteer for another feel good cause, do it! Your participation will make you feel good, and you'll get a chance to share your story with like-minded people who can potentially create more campaign *buzz* for you. The other advantage of doing so is that it will provide you with a learning opportunity to see how other causes go about accomplishing their goals. This can give you better insight into how you might accomplish your goals, as well.

Of course, if you have a family, high school or association reunion coming up, be sure to attend it. This is one of your best avenues for sharing your story. Think about it. No one has seen you in years, possibly decades, and everyone will be asking you "So, what's been going on with you?" or, "What have you been up to these days?" These type of events will provide numerous opportunities to practice your story-telling skills in front of people who have some history with you.

Another option to consider would be to hold individual group sessions, where individual parties who share common interests or associations, can be enlightened all at the same time. For example, you might have a group with your family and extended family. Another could be for friends and another for your peers at your place of employment, educational institution, place of worship, or just about any group that you belong to.

The intention here is twofold. The first objective is to inform the group about your condition, so that they're in the loop. You can tell them that you didn't want to withhold this information from them any longer and that you felt they deserved to know what was going on, should they notice you having a lot of medical appointments. If it's a job related group, do your best to assure your group that your condition will not affect your work—but only if this is true, of course.

The second objective would be to increase their knowledge of the facts surrounding the nation's organ shortage and your need for a living kidney donor. Ask them to share your story and tell them that if they run into someone who might be interested in being your living kidney donor to let you know.

You might be surprised by their responses. Those in attendance might be so moved by your story that they might ask you how they can help or if they could possibly be considered.

If a person responds adversely, thank them for taking the time to listen to your story. They may just be acting out in an attempt to understand your situation better. If they say nothing at all, that's not a bad sign either, as donation is not for everyone— and everyone processes this type of information differently, so give them time.

When it has become clear that someone is not comfortable even talking to you about your situation, or worse, they have overtly told you that they will not help, consider this a gift in disguise. They are telling you not to count on them. Believe me, this is a good thing, even though it feels like you just got punched in the stomach. *Non-participation disclosures* help you identify who's potentially in and who's *not the one*. It's a very efficient way to save you a lot of unhealthy speculation and potential angst.

The mere fact that they had the courage to say they can't do it should be rewarded, so be sure to thank them for their honesty. Adopt this attitude, often taught in sales, and you'll never be impacted by abrupt disclosures.

"Some will, some won't, so what—next!"

183

Remember, living kidney donation is not for everyone. Keep telling your story as often as you can and to as many people as possible. By following these *Donor Magnet®* steps you'll be able to exponentially expand your circle of influence.

If you start early and you're patient enough, you'll be pleasantly surprised to see how many people find themselves attracted to your story.

Step 10: The Power of Intention

The *power of intention* is somewhat synonymous to the principles taught in the law of attraction. *The law of attraction* is a metaphysical belief that states "like attracts like." It is also a theory which states that human perception of both positive and negative thinking, bring about positive and negative results, respectively.

The law of attraction, dates back to the early 1900's during the what was called the *New Thought Movement*. Dakarai Smith, a strong influencer in the *New Thought Movement*, claimed:

"Thought precedes physical form and the action of the Mind plants that nucleus which, if allowed to grow undisturbed, will eventually attract to itself all the conditions necessary for its manifestation."

The highly respected author, Napoleon Hill, directly references *the law of attraction* in his 1928 book, *The Law of Success in 16 Lessons*. In 1937, Hill then published one of his bestselling books, *Think and Grow Rich*, where he explains the importance of controlling one's own thoughts in order to achieve success. He also describes the power our thoughts have and how our thoughts have the ability to attract other thoughts.

Even on Wikipedia, you'll find definitions on the law of attraction relating to how we can attract both positive and negative things into our life based on how we think and what we say. For example, you can either live your life by the following "need based" statement, "I don't have any potential donors right now" and continue to attract more of that lack or need; or you can flip it.

Flipping it would mean that you would restate your belief into a form of abundance, rather than scarcity, like, "I now have several potential donor candidates standing by waiting to be tested," or better yet, "I found my ideal living kidney donor—and I have a wonderful group of very promising potential back up donors standing by." The later accentuates your positive mindset, which, in the law of attraction, has the power to attract more of the same.

An *intention statement* is very similar to the law of attraction, yet it is always in the written form. By creating a written intention statement, you'll be creating a new language for yourself—a language that defines your improved health, happiness and joy.

Start by writing down the top ten things you'd like to manifest in your life, as if you are in the process of achieving them right now. One of your top ten things could be, "I am now attracting excellent living kidney donor candidates into my life."

Once you get comfortable with this first step of *action-based* intention statements that claim *you are in the process of achieving* your goals, you'll need to go back and restate your intentions as if they have already happened. In other words, you'll want to change your action verbs like "attracting" into more powerful verbs. You can do this by restating what you are currently working towards, *as if it has already been achieved.*

For example your statement of: "I am now attracting," would then become, "I now have."

Your intention statement can also include other dreams and goals. You might want to be more open, more curious, more giving or more engaged in the present moment. It can also include your health, happiness, appreciation of and gratitude for the opportunity to live your best life possible.

It doesn't have to be exclusive to your transplant success, though it must be highlighted as your pot of gold.

Keep in mind that your intention statement is a word-based architectural framework of a new language you created for yourself. It can only be written and defined by you. Do not worry that it might sound conceited or arrogant. It only needs to be believed by you first, so it can be emulated in your thoughts and actions.

You will be reading this to yourself and you are reading it often—and the more you think it, write it and read it, the greater the chance it has to attract more of the same.

I know this to be true because it happened to me. One of my most powerful intention statements can be found in the *Charts, Forms & Scripts* section of this book.

All you need to do is dream a bigger dream and then believe that it is not only possible, but that it *already* exists. The mere exercise of writing it out in present tense will create a magnetic field of thoughts to help you attract the reality you're imagining.

So now it's your turn.

Using the principles previously discussed, complete the following actions:

☐ Describe your ideal donor offer. That's right. I'm asking you to get inside the time machine of tomorrow to see your ideal scenario happening right before your eyes.

☐ Now, summon that feeling of immense gratitude while watching this movie play out in your mind.

It shouldn't be too difficult to observe the tender scene where your ideal donor unfolds their offer. Accept this viewing *as if* it were a true accounting of your real life experience.

☐ Repeat this process with your transplant center. Imagine that they just called to tell you that your ideal donor is a great candidate who has been approved to donate to you.

Hear the voice confirming this is true: *"Your donor was approved!"*

☐ Now try to articulate what you envisioned into the written word. Write it out as factual information, rather than a wish or a dream.
This process can be challenging at first, but I assure you that it will be an extremely powerful exercise and well worth the effort.

☐ After you have it written out, print out your first draft. Read the draft and smooth out the rough edges so that it resonates with your heart. Then print out another draft and repeat this refining process until you feel you have it close enough to make it official.

Don't worry about it being perfect, you are free to edit your statement whenever the spirit moves you to do so. (I was moved a lot!)

☐ Now post it on the wall and in several places, so it will be in view upon waking, and while brushing your teeth every morning and before bedtime.

☐ Print a miniature version for your wallet as well.

Top this process off by sending me an email (email: risa@shiftyourfate.com) to describe your success story. Remember to write it as if you already received astounding results from your intention statement.

Be sure to identify all the things you did that helped you attract your ideal donor. Express yourself from a place of joy and gratitude.

Be sure to carbon copy the email you send me to yourself. The mere act of acknowledging that your intention statement is working can turbo-charge its promise back to you. It can be equally powerful to read an email that you previously sent as a statement of fact.

I personally found my intention statement to be the most powerful essential element within my entire success formula.

Undoubtedly, there will be some of you who may feel this process is just too *silly* or completely outside the realm of your structured mind. Give it a go anyway. You'll have nothing to lose but possible regret for not doing so.

Moreover, it would be a shame to underutilized this profoundly promising exercise because of an equally silly judgment or over-rational mind.

Liberate yourself to believe your best opportunity is not only possible—it's happening now. This is the path to limitless potential.

Life-Changing Wisdom Tips

1. Seek to understand what it would be like to offer a selfless gift of such enormous magnitude, before beginning the process of attracting a living kidney donor into your life.

2. When someone offers to be your donor, assume they do not understand the scope of what they offered to do. Your goal is to give them an overview and then get them linked up to unbiased informational sources so you can avoid a conflict of interest.

3. Build your *Donor Recruitment Team.* Invite family members and friends to *partner* with you. You don't have to go it alone! There are people who care about you *(and want to help)* but can't donate. They feel helpless. Give them something to do. Invite them to help you expand your circle of influence.

4. Consider working with a mentor or coach. You can ask an experienced transplant patient to mentor you, or work with a private coach to keep you focused, motivated and on task. *(See Additional Resources for Coaching & Mentoring Information).*

5. Create an Database for outreach and eBlast your scripted story in written word. Be sure to use the tips provided in this chapter and follow email etiquette.

6. Consider using social media, website, blogs, news outlets and message boards to expand your circle of influence.

7. Organize group gatherings and engage in community opportunities to help you meet like-minded people who can share your story. As you volunteer in meaningful ways (outside personal gain), you're more likely to connect to individuals who share altruistic, human kindness values.

8. Dream a bigger dream and write out your dreams as statements that have already come to fruition.

9. Post your intention statements as many places as you can. Keep it within your view and at arm's reach.

10. Remember, likes attract likes. Follow the golden rule. Treat others with care and kindness because it makes you feel good. The more *feel-good* you create, the greater the chance it will come back your way.

11. Believe in this process and prepare to live your best life possible.

"If There Is A Way
To Do Better—Find It!"

– Thomas Edison

Chapter 11: I Think I Found A Donor.

Now What?

Someone has offered to be your donor, and you are not quite sure what to do next. Before we discuss your next steps, lets quickly review a few important facts.

While some CKD patients are lucky enough to have their initial offer be the one that ends up being the only offer they will ever need, it's wise to recognize that things could come up that might deviate from everyone's expectations.

It is best to be cautiously optimistic during this discovery process. Derailments, disqualification, or external influences—even self-realizations, can play havoc with your hopes and dreams.

Imagine for a moment, what a potential living kidney donor's family or friends might say to them when they hear the news. A common response I've heard is, "What? Are you out of your mind? You hardly know this person!" *or* "What about your children or husband's needs some day?"

Comments like these have caused potential donors to end up bowing out gracefully, particularly if they themselves might be thinking: "Is the surgery really as safe as they say it is?" or, "Will I really be able to live a normal life and go back to work in about 3 weeks, like they said?"

What they don't know will hurt you. Your job is to educate them and provide them third party resources so they feel comfortable with the facts. For example, they

193

need to be aware of the fact that kidney disease typically affects *both* kidneys simultaneously?

Their family needs to be aware of the fact that there is little advantage to having an extra kidney in reserve. Kidney disease doesn't discriminate, it affects both your kidneys. It's not often that a spare comes into play, although it can in unilateral trauma or cancer related situations.

It's also helpful to know that kidney donors are handed a *golden ticket*, so to speak, if they ever needed a kidney down the line. It's kind of like a frequent traveler earning premier ranking for all the miles they've traveled. Kidney donors gain *priority status* for "boarding" on the national transplant list; should that unlikely event manifest itself down the line. And while they may not be positioned before the pediatric patients in need, they are as close to the top of the list as any adult could be.

That fact alone can give potential donors and their loved ones tremendous *peace of mind*. It's also reassuring to know that over 110,000 living donors have donated a kidney over the last 23 years and that donor testing is scrupulously evaluated for donor safety. Potential donors are immediately disqualified if it is determined that the nephrectomy (the removal of their kidney) would put them at risk now or in the future. Their loved ones need to know this!

Actually, these are the things I needed to know before I could even wrap my brain around accepting such an offer from a living kidney donor.

Be insistent on linking interested parties up to information sites that have dedicated pages for this type of information. Both you and your potential donor will find this information extremely valuable.

Offer them your nurse coordinator's phone number if you're that far into the process. That way they can ask questions about the transplant center as well. These resources will be a tremendous asset for you and your potential donors and their immediate family.

Donor Testing

After a potential donor suggests that they are ready to move forward, give them the phone number to your Transplant Center's donor desk so that they can officially document their interest in becoming your living kidney donor.

The first thing they will be asked to do is to pass the initial telephone screening. Only the donor can initiate this call. This action documents that the caller is acting on their own volition.

The potential donor's responses to specific health screening questions during that first call determines their eligibility to proceed to testing. The initial call is also an excellent time for potential donors to ask questions of their own.

Those who pass the telephone interview will be asked to wait for a return call for scheduling purposes, or they will receive an itinerary in the mail of preset appointments for their tests. It is best for the donor to speak up about scheduling preferences and work restrictions so that schedulers can take their requests into consideration.

The appointment timeline can take weeks if the donor's schedule isn't flexible, or if they don't request that they'd like the soonest opportunity available.

The potential donor will be asked to provide records on their most recent routine (annual) health maintenance tests (e.g., pap smear, mammogram, prostate, colonoscopy, skin cancer, etc.) and applicable medical clearances for pre-existing conditions, so they can submit the paperwork to the transplant department before beginning their tests.

Potential living kidney donors will most likely be scheduled for various tests, such as:

- Various blood tests:

    - blood type compatibility
    - tissue testing
    - cross-matching
    - antibody screening
    - transmittable diseases

- Urine testing
- Chest x-ray
- EKG
- Screening for kidney function may include:

    - Ultrasound
    - CAT scan
    - MRI, arteriogram

- Screening for liver function
- Screening for heart disease
- Screening for lung disease
- Screening for cancer
- Screening for past-exposure to viral illness

Potential donors will also be assigned an independent donor advocate, *IDA*, who is not part of the transplant patient's medical team. This staff member advocates for the needs and rights and interests of the donor. Their job is to help potential donors understand the informed consent, evaluation process, surgery, recovery and follow up protocols involved. They are also responsible to make sure the donor's decision is completely voluntary and that they do not feel pressured.

Potential donors are also scheduled to meet with both a clinical social worker and psychologist for a psychosocial evaluation, and a surgeon for medical consultation. Once all results from the entire evaluation process are available, they are reviewed by a multidisciplinary committee that decides whether the donor is able to safely proceed with the donation.

Due to strict protocols and guidelines, potential donors are often turned down, so it's wise to have back-up donors to minimize lost time and distractions from disappointment.

Although it seems that these tests would take several weeks—or months to complete—insistent donors have been known to consecutively schedule their appointments and complete their tests in about four days.

Again, think cautiously optimistic. Should your potential donor be disqualified, know that there is actually a hidden blessing beyond your initial disappointment. First off, the potential donor gets a free pass to a super-charged type of health assessment; and secondly, experts confirmed that they were not the best candidate for you.

197

Not such a bad deal, right? Likewise, the center prevents them from putting themselves in harm's way, something that you would never forgive yourself for. All donor disqualifications are hidden blessings in disguise for all parties involved.

There are, however, other deterrents that keep potential donors from qualifying. This comes into play when potential donors are under the impression that they have to be blood-related in order to offer, or be your exact blood type.

As you now know from the information provided to you in Chapter 7, this is not true. Donors only need to have the right blood type to begin the testing process for a direct donation. Even then, as you may recall, *Paired Donation* can bridge the gap in blood type incompatibility through its unique *exchange program* for incompatible donors and recipients. Likewise, *plasmapheresis*, though it is rarely used, can be considered as an option for stripping antibodies from your blood.

Donors may also be concerned that they would be viewed as having a pre-existing condition if they donated, which might cause havoc with their medical coverage. While this is possible, it rarely happens and it appears to be more of a risk with living liver and lung donors, than living kidney donors.

Donors might also be concerned about the amount of time they would have to take off work, since wages, travel and lodging expenses are not covered by the recipients insurance.

When potential donors are not otherwise able to afford the travel, lodging, meals and incidental expenses for themselves and their accompanying person, they may be able to apply for aid from the National Living Donor Assistance Center, *NLDAC*. They will need to prove they have a financial hardship and that they are not able to receive other State or Federal benefits, or reimbursement from the transplant recipient.

The *NLDAC* is provided by the Health Resources and Services Administration, *HRSA*, through a four year cooperative agreement with the University of Michigan and a subcontract with the American Society of Transplant Surgeons, with the intent to reduce financial disincentives to living organ donation. *(Refer to the Reference Section of this book for contact information to learn more about qualifying rules and to access downloadable application form.)*

Donors are also eligible for sick leave, state disability and other coverage under the Family Medical Leave Act (FMLA). Federal employees are eligible for 30 days paid leave, and states like Wisconsin and Georgia have allowed living organ donors to deduct up to $10,000 in expenses from state income tax. There is pending legislation in other states as well.

Donor Surgery & Hospitalization

With over 110,000 living kidney donor surgeries performed to date, the kidney donor removal surgery, known as a nephrectomy, is performed *laparoscopically* using miniature cameras and instruments that are inserted through small dime-size incisions in the abdominal wall. This less invasive procedure offers the donor a potentially quicker and more comfortable recovery. The old standard of using an *Open Technique*, where a significantly larger incision is made, is now considered a thing of the past unless challenging circumstances warrant this approach.

The donor is typically admitted to the hospital the same day of surgery and released within one to three days. The procedure is performed under general anesthesia and the nephrectomy is performed by a transplant surgeon or urological surgical team who are highly trained to separate the kidney from its surrounding structures. The surgeon guides his actions and movements through a viewing monitor which is linked to the camera-assisted instruments used for the procedure.

After the kidney has been separated from its surrounding structures, the kidney is removed through a 3-4″ incision in the mid portion of the lower abdomen. Both the separation and the removal can take from roughly two to four hours, depending on the overall complexity of the surgery.

After the surgery, the patient is monitored for post anesthesia care in a recovery area for blood pressure, heart rate, oxygen levels, temperature, alertness and pain control. The patient is able to eat as soon as completely awake and not showing any signs of nausea or vomiting.

A Foley catheter (a thin, sterile tube inserted into the bladder to drain urine) is typically attached to the donor's bladder, along with an intravenous line for the administration of fluids and pain meds.

After the patient is transferred to their more permanent area of rest and recovery, pain control is typically administered by the donor through a self-directed set-dose button, as needed.

Since the donor could be at risk for developing dangerous blood clots post-surgery, they may be given special compression stockings to prevent them from forming, as well as a medication to prevent clots from occurring.

The donor is encouraged to begin walking within 12 to 24 hours following the surgery. Personal hygiene can begin soon thereafter, if not before. The donor is usually discharged for home recovery after they have met all of the transplant center's post-procedure protocols.

Most donors are allowed to return to work within three weeks, depending on how strenuous their jobs are. All medical costs are covered by the recipient's insurance, so the donor has no out-of-pocket expenses for hospital related expenditures or pre-surgical testing. In other words, there is zero financial impact to the donor from medical expenditures.

Should the donor ever need kidney replacement throughout the rest of their life, UNOS established a provision that allows living kidney donors to be placed towards the top of the waitlist, should that unlikely event occur and transplantation is their wish at that time.

Donor Rest and Time off Work

Once the donor arrives back home after surgery, they may slowly resume their normal daily activities, but not without caution. The biggest mistake that donors make is overdoing normal activities too soon after the procedure. They feel good enough to do more and then find themselves wishing they hadn't.

Most donors are able to return to work after two

to three weeks, depending on their recovery from surgery and the type of job they have. Donors who have a "desk job" *or* who do most of their work by phone or computer, may be able to return to work much sooner than patients with a more physically demanding job.

Regardless of their job, patients are asked to refrain from high impact sports and activities.

While the transplant center is required to report their living donor outcomes for two years, the patient is advised to seek primary care with their own physician, so they can also monitor their progress and keep themselves healthy. Key targets to monitor on an annual basis would be the urinalysis and creatinine level screening.

Donor Risks & Benefits

Of course, any time someone undergoes major surgery there are risks. The most common ones are infections at the incision site and pain immediately following surgery. However, because the procedure is performed laparoscopically, incisions are very small which significantly reduces discomfort and expedites healing. The statistical risk of dying from this type of surgery is very low. According to the National Kidney Foundation's Living Donor Council, the risk of death for living kidney donors is less than 1% (or 0.06%, which is about 1 in every 1700 procedures).

Generally, living donors volunteer knowing these risks because they feel honored to be of service. And the vast majority say they would do it again if they could.

Donors also report a higher quality of life after donation. Perhaps this is linked to feelings of self-worth and purpose-filled achievement as a result of their gift.

There is no scientific evidence in the 50 years of living kidney donations that there are any ill effects to living with one kidney. Within weeks of donation, the remaining kidney swells in size and increases its filtering power (GFR) to match the power of two kidneys. In short, a living kidney donor's remaining kidney ends up becoming a single *turbo-charged* machine—acting at the capacity of two.

Potential donors should also be made aware of the fact that they could be subjected to issues surrounding medical insurability. And, while this is very rare, donors are encouraged to check with their insurance companies to verify their policy.

Before Announcing Intentions

At first glance, a potential donor's enthusiasm about their decision to donate can often work against them if they aren't mindful of their audience. Oftentimes this happens when they are compelled to share the exciting news with their family and friends, before considering how the news might be taken.

It is far wiser for a potential donor to take a mindful pause before blurting out the magnitude of their intentions. The objective here is to build emotional intelligence about how their decision might impact others—that is, others who care deeply for them and would worry themselves sick about their decision.

Family and friends have a tendency to deter living kidney donors from moving forward, and, in their defense, for understandable reasons. They don't want their loved one to be put in harm's way. It's sort of like the *lioness principle*, where the natural instinct is to protect its cubs.

Spouses, family members and significant others can even become angry—or seem a bit jealous at times. These bitter reactions typically show up when the potential donor is observed as someone who hasn't made much of a sacrifice for the family before, yet now is going to do what they believe is the unimaginable with a stranger or someone they barely know.

While a good number of loved ones are moved by the potential donor's intentions, this typically doesn't happen until after they are out of surgery and their safety has been confirmed. For them, it's like being the wife of an Indy 500 racecar driver. All she can see are the dangers upfront, but after the race, she is nothing but excited, proud and celebratory.

Naturally, the donor's family and friends are focused solely on the donor and not your urgent life-threatening needs. This is particularly true when they don't know you. That is why it is so important for your potential donors to frame the delivery of their intentions in such a way that it is more educational and loving, than disrespectful or threatening.

It may be the only way to mitigate the *shock factor* that follows this type of announcement, or an attempt to talk the donor out of their decision. In their view, no matter how routine or safe the surgery claims to be, it is far too dangerous for their loved-one's altruistic quest.

Of course, there's also the element of your potential donor changing their mind at any time—up to and including the day of surgery. So, be mindful of this when you think it's okay to tell other potential donors "No thanks, I already have a donor." It is best not to disclose who's "in" and who's not.

When a potential donor offers to donate to you, your greatest hope is that they have already discussed their intentions with their family and that the jury is "in" and in your favor. Always encourage a potential donor to discuss their wishes with their family, but not without encouraging them to prepare for the process so they can keep negative reactions to a minimum.

If you have an opportunity to help the donor think through the process of how they plan to tell close family and friends, encourage them to role play how they would present their message. Of equal importance, encourage potential donors to imagine how they'd respond to their family and friend's reactions. It's important to be mindful that they are dealing with a highly sensitive topic. This awareness will help them mitigate negative emotions *or* persuasive dissuasion.

Also, encourage your potential donors to schedule a time to present their intentions to their family to prepare themselves for the intensity of the message they will be delivering. Keep in mind that it's one thing to admire stories about others in the media—and quite another for a daughter to tell her mother, or a husband to tell his wife.

Now, imagine that the person the donor is going to donate to is a complete stranger. This could be well considered as *"way out there"* thinking, with thoughts of the potential donor having a *"screw-loose."*

205

Donors should prepare for opposition as an instinctive reaction without being daunted by it. After all, it is a very common way for family and friends to express their care and concern for another. That said, a wise strategy would be to simply expect persuasive dissuasion and view this type of reaction as a normal response.

Above all, they should take the same amount of time to think about how they'll present their message, as they did to make their decision to donate. The key is to imagine what it would be like to be on the receiving end of this type of message. Below you will find some helpful scripts & tips to help potential donors with their donor announcement:

Step 1: Schedule a time to present your intentions

Potential donors should consider presenting their intentions to family members by suggesting a specific time to talk.

For example, they might say, *"I'd like to discuss something important—but I don't want to do it while I'm distracted at work (or driving, or with the kids, etc.).*

Do you happen to have some time this evening, say around 6PM. Maybe we can arrange to have dinner together?"

Step 2: Minimize Distractions & Be Prepared

Once a potential donor has their listener's undivided attention, they should have a script prepared to work from. This will keep them focused and on topic. It's important to minimize distractions and be in a relaxed environment while sharing their decision to donate. (Refer to the example script in the *Forms, Charts & Scripts* section of this book.)

Since this is a lot of information to take in, the potential donor should not be without some type of a cheat sheet at the very least. This will also allow them to take natural pauses throughout the conversation, without forgetting key points.

The goal is to transform the presentation into a conversation so that their audience has enough time to engage and process what they are hearing. The conversation should close with the donor's next steps, so that their audience knows what will happen next.

Before scheduling the presentation, it would be equally wise for potential donors to be prepared for what could be perceived as off-putting reactions or remarks, such as:

1. *"Why would you do such a thing?"*
2. *"What if something happens to you?"*
3. *"What if your remaining kidney fails?"*
4. *"Have you completely lost your mind?"*
5. *"Does the testing also include psychological counseling?"*

Since these reactions can really throw a potential donor off their game, the Q & A below can help the potential donor be more thoughtful and less emotional when responding to individuals who, in essence, are asking for more information.

207

Q: Why would you do such a thing?

A: "Because I want to and I can. I want to help someone now while I'm healthy—and alive. There's a life-threatening organ shortage in this country and I want to do something about it while I can. Sure, I can wait until I pass, but I choose to do both, while I can. A kidney now and a kidney later, along with a few other organs if they'll take them.

Living kidney donors offer patients in need double the lifespan in function, as compared to deceased-kidney donation—and they have to wait years on a list to get one of those. I'd want my kidney to offer maximum quality of life for as long as possible. I also feel it would be a tremendous privilege to spend the rest of my life knowing I did something so amazing to save the life of another human being."

Q. What if something happens to you?

A: "While there's always risk in any surgical procedure, kidney donation is less than 1%! There are far more risky things in the world that I could do, but I choose not to participate in those. This is my choice. The medical screening process is intensive to reduce associated risks. If they see anything that concerns my well-being, they will disqualify me immediately. The surgeons at [center's name] are among the best in the country.

Believe me, I did my homework before I made this decision. I hope you'll give me a chance to tell you all what I've learned, so you'll be less worried. I know you care about me a lot. I appreciate that so much. I hope to make you proud."

Q: What if your remaining kidney fails?

A: "Great question. I was thinking the same thing. Even though a healthy person can live with one kidney just as well as they can with two, if something ever happened to my remaining kidney, I'd be given priority status on the national transplant waitlist. This priority status is given to me because I'm a person who has already donated a kidney to end the wait of another. This is how I'm assured that I wouldn't have to wait either.

Another interesting fact is that statistically, living kidney donors live longer and healthier lives than non-kidney donors do! I can't imagine this affecting my life much more than any other unknown health risk that may come up for me over my lifetime." *For more information on these donor findings visit:

http://www.scienceline.org/2009/03/04/levitan-health-living-kidney-donor-transplant

Q: Have you completely lost your mind?

A: "While I surely understand why you might question my motivation—and that my decision to donate may (admittedly) seem over the top—I assure you I haven't lost my mind.

It's important to me that you understand what brought me to this decision. Information is power, and I hope you'll give me a chance to explain all that I've learned. I care about you, and I'm deeply touched by your concern."

Q: Does the testing for this procedure also include psychological counseling?

A: "Indeed and certainly! In fact, in addition to screening me from head to toe to ensure that I'm healthy enough to donate one of my kidneys, I'll be observed by social workers and a psychologist to ensure I am of sound mind and am emotionally strong enough for this type of procedure. Oh, in case you didn't know, all medical expenses are paid for by the recipient's health insurance."

If the potential donor would prefer to communicate with their friends and family via email or written letter, a template can be found for this purpose in the *Forms, Charts & Scripts* section of this book.

Regardless of how the communication plays out for family and friends of your potential donors, keep in mind that there is also the element of basic logic outside the influences of these relationships.

Your potential donors may also have to deal with their own inner voice that may be telling them, "*Hey, are you sure about this? Wouldn't it be more wise to hold on to both of your kidneys, in case your family ever needs one?"*

It is extremely important that potential donors be educated enough to make an informed decision. Doubts like these must be addressed before the donor calls into the center, otherwise they won't pass the initial screening.

One of the most heartfelt responses I have ever heard to address this feeling of being torn between a good deed today or banking this valorous act for a future family need, was explained to me this way:

"I've decided to do this now because I can and because someone needs my help today. I don't know if I will be needed in the future, or if I will be able to do this in the future. If my family needs a kidney sometime down the line, we can be equally resourceful at that time."

Fortunately, we live in a nation where altruistic people hold a strong desire to serve others. Yet, because government lacks the ability to increase awareness in this particular area of community volunteerism, there are not nearly enough people coming forward. This lack of awareness continues to stifle increased participation.

You, however, can make a difference, just by telling your story. Your story holds a domino effect that can potentially inspire awareness in campaigns around the globe.

Thanks to the benevolence of all the good *Samaritans* making headline news, living kidney donations are touching the hearts (and kidneys) of so many. My dream is that you can help me expand this effort exponentially.

I'm moved when a living kidney donor shows off their mini-scars, as if they were the extra stripes they earned in a battle they so proudly fought. Indeed, it was that and so much more.

So please, I implore you to encourage your potential donors to do their homework before confirming their desires and intentions with you and others. No one needs the extra stress or pressure just because they were overcome with a heroic sense of humanity at the time they said "I can do that!"

Surprisingly, just a couple of hours on the internet is all that is needed to move someone to the next level of contemplation. A short investment for such an important life-altering decision.

From Intention To Offer

Once the potential donor feels they are ready to turn their decision into an offer, they should think once again before proceeding, by processing the following questions:

1. Would it be wiser to run my thoughts and intentions by a spouse or significant other first?

2. Have I thought about how others might respond, so I can be better prepared to explain my motivation?

3. Should I attempt to educate others before making the announcement?

Each answer is: YES, YES and another triple YES!

212

All of these things should be considered with a high degree of emotional intelligence before proceeding to the next step.

Transplant Center Approval

Being an ideal donor isn't just about being healthy or passing all the tests. It's also about being assertive. Unless the potential donor is *All In* and driving the evaluation process, you may both experience irreparable disappointment.

I know of one donor who was ignored for so long, that I seriously questioned if the center was really interested in saving lives. Not all transplant centers realize how fragile your potential donor relationship is. The person on the other end of the phone is your potential donor's first impression of what will follow. If the reception is less than warm or inconsistent, they can easily step aside.

Fortunately, this potential donor was 110% determined to stay in contact with the center. If the donor hadn't stayed in contact with the center, chances are they would have never had the opportunity to be considered for donation, and their intended recipient might have ended up on dialysis.

It's up to you to stay in contact with your potential donors, so that you can encourage them to stay connected with the transplant center. They are the only ones who can ask for updates and progress reports. The transplant center is not allowed to pass donor information on to you. There are strict regulations, confidentiality safeguards and protocols prohibiting the

213

release of donor information to anyone other than the donor.

Which means, if the donor decided to back out, you'd never know it, unless the donor told you. All you might hear, and perhaps only if you asked, is that the donor didn't qualify. Hence, your best barometer is obtained through direct communication with your donor.

Be sure you cultivate a relationship that is trusting, open and inviting, so that you'll never have to wonder what's going on.

Will My Ideal Donor Please Stand Up!

Amazingly, over the course of three years, I attracted over 21 potential donors into my life. Of all 21 good-hearted Samaritans, five were scheduled for testing. Three of the five went through the entire testing process and one of the three repeated some tests just to see if a mistake had occurred. The fourth only did a partial set of tests and then distractions postponed the continuation.

The fifth ended up being the ultimate surprise of my life. That is to say, her offer sent me to the moon and I'm not sure if I returned home yet, it's been such a high. She did her homework, went through all the tests and passed with flying colors.

She's known to me as the amazing *MAKster*, and as you will soon discover, she is a truly amazing human being.

MAK's Blessing

On June 8, 2010, I received a beautiful and highly functioning kidney from one of the most extraordinary people I've ever met. Her name is Melissa, but my husband and I call her *The MAKster.*

I was fortunate to meet Melissa at the transplant center where I had been evaluated and approved. From the moment she walked through the door, she had me at "Hello." I couldn't really explain that special feeling at the time, but Melissa describes it as a *kindred spirit* sort of connection we shared.

Kindred spirits indeed, as we matched on 5 out of 6 antigen markers—a score that true blood sisters should get!

The event which led to our connection occurred after all my potential donors had been disqualified, and I felt a need to better understand the donor qualification process. I requested a meeting and a woman named Melissa was scheduled to speak to me. I found myself exhilarated by this woman's presence and very grateful that someone in management would take the time to meet with me.

As luck would have it, I was granted the privilege to meet with her three more times over the course of five months. During those sessions, we discussed the need to improve CKD patient education while sharing examples of how the living kidney donor evaluation process was somewhat fragile. We agreed that the process could be confusing for both potential donor and recipient.

After our meetings I would return home to reflect on my own process. Along the way I decided to review my donor journal to see if I had overlooked anything that could be holding me back. Then it hit me. While I had been open to receiving several donor offers, I had not fully focused on attracting my "ideal" donor offer.

It was time to walk my talk and put more **PEBO®** into my intention, so I could Proactively Empower my Best Outcome. I immediately went to my computer and opened up a new document. It all felt so natural. The most profound words appeared on the screen, though I can't recall instructing my fingers to strike the keys below them. It was like approaching my driveway without recalling the road that took me home.

The piece was entitled: *"Will My Ideal Donor Please Stand Up!"* It was a document that subsequently became my renewed *intention statement*. In this statement, I affirmed the exact month that my ideal donor would appear and all the particulars surrounding the surgery.

I also confirmed the donor was already approved by the Mayo Clinic's Selection Committee and that both donor and recipient were in ideal health to undergo the surgery. I described how successful both surgeries were and I spoke of expedited donor healing, the ease of recovery and the impact this procedure would have on the world. (See Written Intention Statement Example in the *Forms, Charts and Scripts* section of this book).

The more I typed, the more my thoughts and feelings flowed. While each and every word held intense personal meaning, the most profound inspiration occurred after I described how my body would embrace this new part of me.

I pledged in writing that I would care for my new kidney as if it were my own—like a mother cares for her newborn or how creatures of nature instinctively care for their off-spring.

I can't really explain it, but this "act as if" mindset made me feel as though I had literally cracked the code to *shift* my fate.

The more I declared my intentions and beliefs, the more I believed that anything was possible and that everything was happening just the way it should—and for all the right reasons.

The first inkling of my intentional efforts unveiled itself on Easter Sunday, just three days after the birth of my written intention statement. An older gentleman—an Englishman who identified himself as Dr. Jim—called to see if he could be tested. He was 70 years of age (age range for the donor is from 18-65) and his blood-type was incompatible, but he was willing to explore paired donation possibilities.

Then, the following day—just four days after I completed my written intention statement, a dental assistant whom I had never met, gestured that she might like to see if she could be my donor too. The offer occurred while she was loading a digital sensor into my mouth to capture a few radiographic images. (Donors appear in the darnedest places!) She too was blood type incompatible, but interested in learning more.

Then, exactly 10 days after writing my intention statement, the most unbelievable of all offers manifested itself right before my eyes. It was an offer from Melissa. And while you might be saying to yourself, "Gosh that's so wonderful," what I'm about to tell you about Melissa will help you understand why her offer was so remarkable, and why I was so astounded.

First, Melissa is not a manager, she's Mayo Clinic's Operations Administrator and a registered nurse.

And, if that wasn't amazing enough, she's also responsible for the entire Transplant Center, as well as the divisions of Nephology, Hepatology and Infectious Diseases. She manages over one hundred staff members—nurse coordinators, doctors and surgeons report to her!

Melissa's spirit is even more compelling when you learn about the significance of her motivation to become a living organ donor. As she tells the story, fifteen years ago while working at another hospital as a transplant nurse coordinator, she had an epiphany. It occurred when the family of a dying baby, who was soon to be taken off of life support, refused organ donation consent—consent, that could have saved the life of another baby down the hall.

That night two babies died. And that night, Melissa became an ardent organ donation proponent. After observing that experience, Melissa made a decision to donate an organ to someone, someday, while she was still living.

Of course, I had no idea that when she was telling me this that the someday could be now, and that the someone could be me. After sharing her history with me, there was a brief pause and then my heart was overtaken by some of the most surreal expressions a CKD patient could ever imagine. She said, "I have given this a lot of thought Risa. I'm your blood type. I'm healthy and the perfect age—and I have two healthy kidneys. I've decided to be your kidney donor."

I'm pretty sure I stopped breathing at that point, I don't recall much other than the fact that she literally took my breath away. I was in a state of shock and deeply moved, all at the same time. Tears welled my eyes and my body became weightless, as if I was soaring with an angel—a real-life *living* kidney donor angel and her name is Melissa!

In that moment, I silently acknowledged to myself that my intention statement was unfolding right before my eyes, and doing so with the most unanticipated candidate I could have imagined.

It all felt like a dream—and then it occurred to me, it was a dream—a dream come true! It was the *dream* that I had written as a *reality* in my intention statement. It was like watching the beginning of the movie play out from those scenes I had created in my mind, without knowing who the actors were outside my own role.

It was both exhilarating and mysteriously wonderful all at the same time. It was April. She was my blood type, she knew exactly what she had just volunteered to do. I can't explain why, but for some reason, I had no doubt she'd be approved. Somehow I knew, with the same certainty our earth will rotate around the sun from a gravitational force between them, that my life would never be the same.

And, let me tell you, it hasn't! With vibrant health and a .8 Creatinine —something I haven't seen in decades—I am one of the luckiest girls alive!

Surely, now, you can understand why her offer was so special and why my husband and I endearingly call Melissa *The MAKster*. After all, she gave me *MAK*, the nickname I gave my precious new kidney, which is an acronym that so fittingly represents **M**elissa's **A**mazing **K**idney.

Ironically, neither one of us ever had children, yet Melissa tells me that she feels like a proud mother. I too, feel like I am a blessed parent, who just adopted the most precious child in the world. Words cannot accurately describe the gratitude I feel for *The* MAKster through the blessing she gave me—and the health *MAK* gives me every single glorious day of my renewed and most vibrant life.

Melissa's offer was one of the most profound surprises of my life and her gift will always be cherished for the value it brings by giving me quality of life and renewed health.

On June 8th of every year we rejoice in the celebration of my renewed health in what Melissa coined as our *KidneyVersary®*—and what an extraordinary celebration it has become.

You too can celebrate your own *KidneyVersary*. All you need to do is pledge to become a *PROactive* kidney patient, so you too can live your best possible life. If you break it down to its simplest form, you have nothing to lose. There's no pills, diets or harmful side effects.

Give it a try. If you don't feel it's for you, you can always go back to your life as you know it today. That is, if that would be your choice after considering what you now know from the information in this book.

It's far easier to verbalize what you intend to do, than it is to actually do what you intended. But now, you can use the pearls between these pages as your breadcrumbs, to ensure you'll never lose your way, even if you do get distracted from time to time.

Remember, it's not a matter of *if* you believe you will ever develop complete renal failure, it's a matter of experiencing failure of a completely different kind. Failure to do something, while you had a chance to do something, like change your fate.

Please don't fall into that trap by looking the other way or saying "on another day." Don't subject yourself to heartbreaking and shameful regret.

Accept the fact that you may lose your remaining renal function someday—if you haven't already, and make up your mind that your life matters.

If this book fell into your hands—before your need for dialysis—you have an excellence chance of dramatically changing your fate. A chance most CKD patients rarely get. Now that you know you have this opportunity, and you now have the tools to impact your future, initiate the process now!

All you need to do is choose a *Proactive Path* with powerful intention—and you'll soon be on your way to achieving the most fulfilling life you ever imagined.

Think BIG.

Dream BIGGER

Apply the Life-Changing Wisdom from this book to

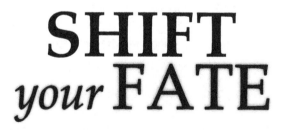

SHIFT
your FATE

& Secure Your Best Life Possible!

Life-Changing Wisdom Tips

1. Educate potential donors and provide them resources so they know exactly what's involved. This helps them make an informed decision while communicating their intentions to loved ones.

2. Encourage your potential donors to be assertive when interacting with the transplant center, so they stay connected and in the loop. Keep your relationship open and trustworthy, so they will keep you in the loop too.

3. Help your donor understand the importance in preparing for their announcement to donate with loved ones. Preparation should include role-playing. Good preparation will mitigate contention and keep negative emotions at bay.

4. Encourage donors to discuss their intentions with loved ones before they call the transplant center, but not without considering #1,#2 and #3 above.

5. Never underestimate the power of the written word through written intention statements. Position your dreams in the reality that they will become, but do it as if they have already happened to elicit manifestation.

6. Think BIG. Dream BIG and then dream a BIGGER dream.

7. You have the chance to change your fate. Do it!

8. Use this life-changing wisdom to shift your fate—and prepare to live your best life!

"Life is a Celebration of the Soul.
It's Time to Celebrate."

Donors & Recipients Tell Their Story

Living Kidney Donor Stories

Living Kidney Donor Story #1

There was never a question in my mind about donating one of my kidneys. I had watched Ryan, the love of my life, struggle with dialysis for years before receiving his first deceased-donor kidney, which was transplanted back in 1997. When it was nearing the end of its term in 2007, I knew I was supposed to be his donor this time around.

Suddenly, Ryan's life took a turn for the worse when it was threatened by a deadly viral infection he had contracted. I guess I could have been diverted then too, but it didn't stop me then and I never looked back or changed my mind. If anything, it made me even more determined to move full steam ahead with my intentions. When he was able, I would donate. That's all I knew and that's all I thought about after almost losing him to the effects of the serious virus he contracted and the damage it had caused.

Ryan survived three surgeries to follow, but the trauma from the procedures positioned him back on dialysis. His transplanted kidney was no longer functioning at an acceptable level. I noticed a considerable difference in Ryan after his hemodialysis appointments, which he religiously endured three times a week. Unlike the Peritoneal dialysis he had been on before his transplant, this one really took a toll on his body. I observed his body deteriorating, both physically and mentally. He lost weight, became depressed and his thinking became cloudy. He also slept a lot at night and napped often

224

during the day. It was time to ramp up the process and finish my testing!

It took about a year's time, from start to finish, to be tested, retested, evaluated, re-evaluated and then, finally approved. For whatever reasons, I had no worries going into this. After all, I was told that if I ever had a problem with my remaining kidney after donation, I would receive preferential treatment and be positioned up towards the top of the list. And, while that was reassuring to know, I had already decided that I was going to donate my kidney to Ryan regardless. And on March 5th 2009, that's exactly what I did.

I recall us both being positioned in adjacent rooms, dressed in our matching gowns, caps and booties. We used hand signals to express our love and appreciation for one another. And, then, in the blink of an eye, we were off to the O.R.

I remember my surgeon greeting me with, "It's a beautiful day!" and the next thing I knew, the surgery was behind me. Of course, the first instinct was to check to see how Ryan was doing. I was told he was doing extremely well. I was so relieved and pleased with the news. Eventually, we were able to send several text messages to each another, with passionate and intended redundancy. Our three most favorite words "I love you!" never seem to get old or trite. We knew what we meant and that's all that mattered.

While in separate rooms and on separate floors, we felt even closer than ever before. Yet, within 30 hours' time, I was discharged to go home. I couldn't imagine going home without Ryan. Who would keep an eye on him, like I would, I thought to myself? With no reassurance in sight, I took it upon myself to sneak up to his room after I was discharged and I camped out on the couch for the remaining 5 days of his stay.

225

While this isn't something I would recommend donors do, I wasn't going to have it any other way! They'd have to try to kick me out, and I'd be kicking and screaming all the way. If it was going to happen, it would happen over my dead body and I knew the center had certain standards they have to report regarding donor survival rates, so I was pretty sure my "fort" was secured.

From the moment I set eyes on Ryan, I could see his color was back and his spirit was shining. His surgeon even told us both that the surgeries were a glowing success and that we were obviously meant for one another. In fact, we were a perfect antigen match!

It's such an honor to donate a kidney while still living. Giving life is one of the greatest rewards in the world. And, while donating at the end of life is equally honorable and something I plan to do as well, giving while living, is on a plateau of its own. Simply put: I did something while I was alive so I could see the prize inside another. Life just doesn't get any better than that!

And, while Ryan shares his gratitude with me daily, it is I who feels the most thankful. I'm thankful that he never gave up and that he accepted my gift, for he now holds the spirit of not only my heart, but now my kidney too!

Living kidney donation has allowed me to do so much more than just comfort Ryan in his time of need. It allowed me to make his dreams come true. Most of all, it allowed me to feel helpful at a time in which I had felt so helpless.

My gift also makes me feel like an exceptional human being. It's a transcendent experience, that is unique, immeasurable and by far, the highest honor I have ever achieved in my entire lifetime. And, while some may argue that

226

the recipient is the only one who receives the gift, I feel equally privileged.

If I can leave a message for those who may be intrigued by my story, or who may be contemplating living kidney donation for themselves, I say: "Don't be afraid, my friend." Sure, I experienced real pain after surgery, and any surgery would have its risks. Yet, the risks in living donation are less than 1% — and the pain I experienced was like the pain a hero might feel after fighting a battle to end the war.

It's a victorious inconvenience that can be controlled with some medication, rest and relaxation. Not such a bad deal for someone who needs to rest more often anyway. Truth be known, my biggest challenge was keeping myself from overdoing. Perhaps that gives you an idea of how bad I actually felt!

Like Nike® says, "Just Do It!" You will feel the same with one kidney, as you did with two--only spiritually better after donation! Honestly, it's an experience of a lifetime that unexpectedly unveils the type of hidden greatness you never knew you had before.

I now live my life with purpose, respect and admiration of this accomplishment - and in pure gratitude that my love of my life, now has a life worth living for. And all of this for just sharing my spare. I'm a living kidney donor. You can be one too!

-Kim P.

Living Kidney Donor Story #2

In January 2008, at the Mayo Clinic in Phoenix Arizona, I proudly donated my left kidney to a friend. I lived a fairly typical life up until then and have continued to live a normal one since. I live in Kansas City, MO with my husband,

Patrick, and my three children, (two at the time of the transplant.) I have two older sisters and lots of amazing friends. I am active in my church, and I like to do various kinds of art. I also love to sing.

I have worked in non-profit my entire career and I am inspired by helping people find their voice and get empowered to fight back against the struggles they are facing. That's how I met Dean, my kidney transplant recipient.

We got to know one another through my work with the Polycystic Kidney Disease (PKD) Foundation, a small nationally recognized non-profit, where I helped develop and then manage their National Walk. Dean, the lead coordinator and chief volunteer for the Phoenix Walk and I worked together while coordinating the event he ran in his region.

Whenever this subject comes up about me being a living kidney donor, people want to know if we are amazing life-long friends. I guess people expect a dramatic movie script — something astonishing that inspired me to donate a body part. But for me, it just wasn't that dramatic. It was a simple moment where God whispered the idea in my ear. I just happened to listen and say yes.

It all began the day I arrived in Phoenix for a marketing meeting with a local TV station. Dean accompanied me. The meeting was a success and we headed back to the airport, chatting away as the rain fell around us.

The conversation about his need of a new kidney was just a casual sidebar to our ride back to the airport. To see him, you'd never imagine that this kind, personable, fun to be around guy, who was young, good-looking and fit, was nearing renal failure and was fighting for his life. He spoke of a donor that was being tested on his behalf who looked promising. Yet, for no real apparent reason, a thought popped into my head, "It's not her; it's supposed to be me."

I didn't say anything at the time and when we arrived at the airport, we said our goodbyes and I flew home. The first thing I did was share my thoughts with my husband. My husband smiled and said, "I think that's awesome, honey. Whatever you want to do, I'll support it." He was used to supporting a lot of crazy stuff with me, I guess. From what I understand, this is not the typical response at all.

A week later I emailed Dean to see how it was going. He said his donor had been kicked out in the final round of tests, so his search was back on. I instantly replied that I'd like to be tested.

Next was a phone call to his transplant center, to see if I could pass the telephone interview and medical history.

I cleared that hurdle. Next up was blood matching. They mailed me a kit, I had blood drawn in Kansas City and shipped it over-night to Phoenix. If our blood "got along" I'd have to fly back to Phoenix for about a week of extensive tests. It wasn't until the blood test came back that I told the rest of my family. That was a little trickier than telling my husband.

My mother's first concern was my health. She asked a lot of "what if?" questions, concerned about future health issues for me. I let her tell my dad, who was equally concerned, but I let her address all the questions. My dad and I were very close and it's not that he wasn't interested or concerned. Quite the opposite. I think it was just too hard for him to talk about.

My oldest sister was similarly concerned for my well-being, but she was instantly supportive. She understood the God-whisper I spoke of. She said, "Leigh, some people go on huge shopping sprees, some do extreme sports, some drink too much... You push back against the unhappiness and stress in your life by doing nice things for other people. Not a bad way to deal with stuff."

Telling my other sister wasn't so easy. One of her first questions was if one of the tests was a psych test! Which indeed it was, and I passed – so I am certifiably sane and I have the test results to prove it. Though we got a great laugh out from those discussions, her real concern was, "What if something went wrong?" She was worried that I might be unable to emotionally handle it. We talked it through and I assured her I'd be Okay.

Of course, I had to clear it at work. Working for a kidney organization certainly made the request for time off to donate a kidney to a constituent a lot easier for me than for someone else, but I was still pretty nervous about telling them. They were instantly supportive and said I'd get all the time I needed – even made sure I got my full salary versus the disability pay for the time I was off. What a blessing.

The real challenge came in talking about it. I did not want to tell others at work and I swore my superiors to secrecy. I didn't want any other staff members to feel any pressure, to be made to feel the hard work they did every day for all our kidney patients was somehow "less". Thankfully, they honored my wishes and allowed me to tell my co-workers when I was ready – the week before I left for the transplant.

But I am getting ahead of myself here. After the blood test – which I passed with flying colors, we had to schedule a week in Phoenix for full tests. It was set up for the week of my birthday, in early November. I seemed to sail through all the tests, though it was a long 4 days. There was lots of back and forth, a dozen different doctors and a lot of peeing in a bottle. My last day in Phoenix before flying home, Dean and I had a *toast while we watched a beautiful sunset and I just knew it was going to happen.*

Thanksgiving week I got the phone call announcing my approval. In January of 2008, I flew back to Phoenix and checked into Mayo Clinic and donated a kidney. A week later I flew home to Kansas City; six weeks later I was back at work on a full schedule.

Now almost four years post nephrectomy, I'm healthier than I have been in a long time. Life rolls on as usual. I said farewell to my father in June of 2010 and on November 23rd of that same year, I gave birth to Thomas Wilson, an amazing baby boy weighing 7 pounds and 10 precious ounces. I never had any complications during pregnancy and having just one kidney caused no issues whatsoever, proving once again that a living kidney donor can go on to live a normal, healthy life.

I not only live a healthy life, I live a very full life. Together with my husband, I am raising our three kids – one teenager (need I say more?), a very precocious and determined pre-teen daughter, and a joy-filled, busy baby.

I now work at more-than-a-full-time job with a company that specializes in helping a number of charities find their voice and fulfill their mission through events and fundraising. I also run a large Outreach Committee at my church and put on an annual Block Party for the underprivileged neighborhood where our church resides; we welcome about 300 visitors each year.

I am also a lead member of our church Praise Team, which allows me to pursue my passion for singing, for all the right reasons. And, I write a blog that is all about throwing some good out into the world. Yes, life is full, and my life is blessed and I try every day to be a blessing.

What I did was really not a big deal in my life at all, though I count it among the greatest blessings in my life – second only to giving birth to my kids and hiking the Grand Canyon. It is hard to put into words, but the feeling of knowing you just did a good thing, wanting nothing in return, can't be matched.

I am not sure of the ripple effects that the whole experience had, but I know they are there. I just listened to the voice that said "do it" and then said "YES!" I took a few weeks off and then went back to my life. The only lasting thing for me is a few small scars on my stomach and a keener ear for the voice in my head that sometimes suggests I do something kind. For me, I believe it is the voice of God, whispering in my ear, giving me an opportunity to be used by Him for something grander than I could ever manufacture on my own.

Sometimes I ignore the whisper. I am sure that sometimes I am making far too much of my own noise to hear it at all. But when I can shut out my voice and listen to His... Wow, what a blessing.

Not everyone is called to donate a kidney, but I believe many more are ready to answer YES, if they were made aware of the need. If more of us answered the call, far fewer lives would be lost to kidney disease.

Everyone is called to do something. Everyone has a unique and special thing to throw out into the world and far too many of us ignore that inner voice and miss the opportunity.

So my question for you is, "What is He whispering in your ear today? Will you listen and say YES?"

-Leigh R.

Living Kidney Donor Story #3

I was signed up to be a donor on my driver's license. I was never exposed to someone needing an organ, so I never thought about donating an organ while I was alive.

I was working at a vitamin store at the time and one of my favorite customers called me and was upset because she wanted to donate her kidney to her daughter who needed one, but she had been ruled out because of her age. Never giving it a second thought, I offered to donate my kidney to her.

As I suspected, I received some opposition from my husband, but I didn't let that change my mind. I felt God had called me to do this. My husband came around within time like I thought he would eventually do, but I see now that communicating to your family requires well deserved forethought.

We started the process, which was a lot of trips to the Mayo Clinic and a lot of waiting. Thank God I was committed to this process because there were lots of hiccups. When they did an ultrasound of my kidney the doctors saw my left kidney was okay and the right one had an anomaly on it.

They came back to me and my recipient and said, they were not ruling me out to donate but that I would only be used as a last resort. If my donor could find a more suitable match it would be better. My recipient was having her native kidneys removed, which would have made the surgery longer and more intense. They didn't want to complicate the situation by having to deal with the anomaly on my right kidney.

I was very disappointed with the news and I started questioning God whether I was really supposed to donate. I felt very happy and disappointed at the same time when my recipient found another donor. I was so happy for her, but I

233

started questioning if I really was supposed to do this.

Several months after my recipient's surgery I got a call from her asking if I would still like to donate. I said yes. She introduced me to a woman who was nearing dialysis and in desperate need. Because it had been over a year from the time I started testing, I had to start over with all the tests. Lots of trips and lots of waiting.

They still saw the anomaly and finally decided to take the case back to the committee. After several weeks of back and forth, conflicting opinions from the committee and numerous delays, I was officially approved to donate.

On February 10, 2011 I met my recipient at Mayo Clinic and we prayed together before we were admitted. The whole experience was so amazing. Both surgeries were a complete success, and now my recipient's life has been greatly improved and my life was barely impacted from the brief discomfort I experienced.

It has been a year since the surgery and I feel so blessed that God chose me to save another person's life. I am also grateful that I stuck to my intention to stay-the-course, even when I was given detours along the way. As it turned out, the anomaly they were so concerned about was not as bad as they imagined it to be. Between our prayers - and her amazingly talented surgeon - it didn't challenge the success of the surgery whatsoever!

I recently met a man who desperately needs a kidney. He said he didn't want his kids to donate. I told him he was depriving his kids of a blessing and the most wonderful gift of love they might ever experience in their life. I told him that they have a chance of saving their dad's life. And, while their life would not change, his would dramatically change for the better.

I hope anyone intrigued with the possibility of donating, or recipients who are concerned about accepting such a gift, talk to those of us who have donated. I have never met a donor who regretted having done so, myself included.
GOD BLESS.
- Pam S.

Living Kidney Donor Story #4

Personally, I had never really thought about organ donation other than checking that box on my driver's license. However, one day in January 2013, an email came out from the Cave Creek Unified School District, where my two children attended school. Their elementary-school principal, had polycystic kidney disease and needed a kidney.

Her children and siblings were tested for the disease and none were a match. This was when I felt the first nudge.

I called the principal's assistant and discovered a lot of people had already called in and several were undergoing testing. A few months later, however, I discovered they had not yet found a match. This is when I knew I was the one.

I contacted Mayo Clinic and began a battery of tests, including a blood work up for tissue typing and cross-matching. On September 3rd I was medically cleared to be a living kidney donor. I wasn't surprised. I was excited.

We picked the date — January 7, 2014 since we had to take a month off work. We had an understanding that if it became medically necessary for her health, we would go in sooner.

235

The surgery went great. I stayed in the hospital for one night, and Nancy stayed two.

My recovery was smooth and I had a little pain and discomfort the first week. I was mostly just tired. I weaned myself off the pain pills as soon as I could. Emotionally, I was on a high.

We were both overwhelmed by the outpouring of love and support from the community. Notes, flowers, gift cards for dinners and handmade cards from entire classes at the elementary school poured in. A school song was even written and social media exploded with well-wishers. It was both humbling and amazing.

Post-transplant, we are both back to work and living amazing lives. What's more, the entire experience has changed me. It made me realize just how important it is to give to others in this life. Life is a journey, and we are called to be our best selves and love our neighbors.

This donation allowed me to give the gift life while I was still living. If you're ever lucky enough to be a donor match —just do it. I did, and have not regretted it for a second. And, while I'm sure that my recipient feels like she was the one blessed — I'm the one who feels like the winner.

-Kati W.

A Donor's Mother's Perspective:

I am a mother of a child who donated a kidney to a stranger. At first, I struggled over my daughter's decision. (Mothers are supposed to protect their daughters and keep them out of harm's way.) I could have benefited greatly from another mother's perspective. In the spirit of sharing my journey to help empower other mothers, I wrote this open letter.

Dear Loved One of a Potential Living Kidney Donor:

When my daughter announced she wanted to donate a kidney to a stranger, I was of course concerned. Yet I wasn't as concerned about the surgical outcome as I was for my daughter's future. I thought, "What if she ever had kidney failure herself?" While I've always trusted my daughter's judgment, I couldn't help but ask if she was sure this was something she really wanted to do. She assured us that she had researched the process diligently and that she was 100% confident about her decision.

She expressed her passion for what she believed was a calling to serve. She shared the details of the procedure, highlighting the safeguards that were in place to protect living kidney donors. She also conveyed a tremendous amount of faith in her medical team, which put my mind at ease.

The real turning point for me occurred when I shifted my focus towards my belief in the **Golden Rule**. I simply put myself in the place of the parent with a child in need. Then I asked myself, "How could I stand in the way of my daughter's calling to save someone's life?" Then I knew the answer. *I surely wouldn't want someone to stand in the way if my child needed such a gift, so how could I stand in the way of another mother's child?*

I'm so proud of my daughter and I'm deeply moved by the spirit of her kindness. I'm equally honored to be the mother of such a gifted and selfless soul.

Sincerely,
Diane

Transplant Recipient Stories

Transplant Recipient #1 — Paired Donation
Involving A 22 Person Chain

My grandmother died at age 56 of Polycystic Kidney Disease (PKD) and my mother died at age 57. I will turn 59 this year. Thanks to a remarkable young man named Matt Jones along with my husband's amazing generosity, I am eagerly looking forward to a long and healthy future with my grandchildren. I'd like to share the extraordinary set of events leading up to my kidney transplant at Banner Good Samaritan Hospital in Phoenix.

This may sound like a story about kidneys, but it's really a story about heart. In 1975 when my husband, Ron, and I were married, he gave me his heart and we exchanged the traditional vows in sickness and in health. Who could foresee how this would actually play out?

In 1982, I was diagnosed with PKD – distressing news for our young family. Ron decided that he would give me one of his kidneys when the time came. Other than monitoring my blood pressure and adapting to a heart-healthy diet (something we all can benefit from), we channeled all our energy into raising our two boys.

By the end of 2006, my kidney function had dropped below 20%. We began the final testing for a transplant. At the last minute, we received some devastating news – it turned out that I had developed antibodies to Ron's antigens during my two pregnancies. We were incompatible and Ron would not be able to give me a kidney. Thus began the roller coaster ride of navigating our way through an unfamiliar health care system.

We found out about Paired Donation and felt a surge of optimism. We assumed that all we needed was to find another couple in a similar situation. Ron would donate his kidney in exchange for me receiving one. Seems easy, right? Then we encountered two major obstacles. There is no national data base for live donor matches and no transplant center in Phoenix, including Banner, was tied into a regional database. Secondly, we were told there was only a 2% chance for a successful match within each regional program--not very good odds.

Dr. Alfredo Fabrega, head of Banner's Kidney Transplant program, suggested that we contact the University of Toledo Medical Center in Ohio. Dr. Michael Reese had come up with the novel idea of using an altruistic donor to start a kidney chain, thus increasing dramatically the odds of making successful donor pairings.

After numerous tests, it turned out that I was a perfect match with Matt Jones, an amazing young man from Petoskey, Michigan. Matt had a big kidney and an even bigger heart. Matt, a burly young man and father of five, told me that he wanted to give me one of his kidneys. He said, "I want nothing in return except that Ron pay it forward." When I asked him why, he said, "I want to do something my kids can look at and remember me by. I want to leave a legacy."

Ron and I were very fortunate to have the rich bonding experience of meeting Matt in person the week before my surgery. We were all a little nervous, and the doctors cautioned us that it was not the normal protocol. However, we all wanted to meet and since then, he has become part of our extended family. We have shared hugs, tears and, of course, a kidney.

We also discovered a cosmic connection with Angi – the then 32 year-old woman who was to receive Ron's kidney. We were in Toledo in 2007 for Ron's clinical work-up on June 21st and celebrated our 32nd anniversary that evening. The next day, we met Angi for the first time – on her 32nd birthday! She was born the day after we were married. If Ron had any doubts

239

*about giving his kidney to someone else, they disappeared after meeting Angi. He left saying, "I don't care if my kidney lasts six months, six years or the rest of her life. This is the right thing to do." The silver lining of our situation was the opportunity to become part of something much larger and more impactful in the world of organ transplants – the first **Pay-it-Forward** donor chain.*

Angi had been on dialysis for over 12 years and had experienced several life-threatening events. Now she's in college, studying to become an ultra sound technician. Her mother, Laurie, continued the chain by donating to another woman two months after Angi's surgery. "There's nothing better," Laurie said, "than watching someone's life improve."

Back to my transplant story — on July 18, 2007 Matt donated his left kidney to me. In spite of him "feeling like he had been hit by a truck," Matt insisted on coming up to see me the day after our surgeries, and we had a brief but joyful reunion. He made an incredible personal sacrifice to give me back my health, all from the goodness of his heart.

I had my surgery on Wednesday and was discharged on Sunday. The next day, Ron left for Toledo to continue the donor chain. Although it was difficult to say goodbye, we both felt very good about the next step in our journey. We became the first people in the United States to start a non-simultaneous transplant chain. Amazingly, everyone in our chain has fulfilled their personal commitment to pay forward their kidney over the past 4½ years – a true testament to the spirit of giving.

I found out later about Ron's final conversation with his surgeon before heading into the operating room. The doctor told him, "You are healthy and there is no medical reason for you to undergo surgery. Your chance of death is 1 in 3,000 – if you don't want to proceed, your reasons will be kept confidential."

Ron's reply was, "That risk is bigger than I want to take—unless you can guarantee me that if something happens during surgery, you will do everything you can to harvest all my organs, including my heart..." That was so typical of Ron – his heart is always in the right place, but his timing is sometimes a bit off. Who wants their doctor in tears before starting surgery.

Well, as you all know, this story has a great ending. Five years later, we are all healthy and enjoying life to the fullest. We recently met for a weekend get-together on Mackinac Island in Michigan. Last April, Matt and his wife, Meghan, came to Phoenix for a visit. While they were here, we decided to get tattoos to honor our commitments to each other. Matt wanted to "replace" his donated kidney so he had a life-like kidney tattooed on his left hip. Meghan and I had **Life is Good** flowers done on our feet, and Ron had a **Life is Good** tattoo on his calf. These provide a constant reminder to all of us that every day is a gift.

-Barbara B

Transplant Recipient Story #2

I lost my renal function due to a genetic disorder that I inherited from my dad, known as PKD. I was told I didn't have the gene when I tested as a teenager, so you can imagine the extent of my shock to learn otherwise. This was a disease that took my father's life in his early forties and I was in my late 30's at the time. I was certain I was on the same road of no return.

It was not long after my diagnosis that I was forced onto dialysis (1993). Peritoneal dialysis became my life for nearly 3 years. This was a process that required 2 liter bags of

241

special fluid that would hang on an IV pole above my head, with an IV connected to a catheter which was surgically implanted in my abdomen to access the internal cavity.

I was required to do this 4 times a day, and the process took about 30 minutes from start to finish. Infection control was critical during this procedure to avoid possible infection from contaminated hands and air. I wore a surgical mask and gloves, but only after washing my hands repeatedly.

The fluid remained in my body for several hours until it was time to drain. It felt like I was carrying an extra 7 pounds of fluid in my belly. When it was time to drain, the fluid drained into an empty bag, from the outflow tube on my catheter, which was then connected to a empty bag, now positioned for gravity flow on the floor. There was no reprieve. After draining, I was to repeat the process of filling my belly with a fresh bag of fluid and the process started anew.

Unfortunately, even though I was extremely diligent about cleanliness and sterility, I experienced not one, but three episodes of serious, life-threatening infections. After miraculously surviving all three, I now understand how these dialysis associated risks would be extremely challenging for anyone to avoid.

While on dialysis, I found myself bound to a restrictive life style and schedule, which challenged my emotional wellbeing. I dropped into a deep state of depression and could only maintain my purpose in life through therapy and medication.

I was blessed with a kidney transplant from a cadaver kidney in April 1997, after waiting on the transplant list for over three years. (Today the wait in my area is nearly nine!) My new kidney lasted for 11 strong years and most likely would have lasted another year, if not for another infection I acquired that led to a few life threatening events, including a triple bypass surgery.

Surviving both the events and their required surgeries, I found myself back on dialysis, except this time it was hemodialysis (for 9 months). This time, I had a small catheter in my upper chest. I didn't have to have a new fistula in my arm because the love of my life, Kim, already started testing on my behalf. And, while I can't deny it was really rough this second time around on dialysis, I had a completely different mental state of contentment in the knowing that my wait would be shorter and the outcome would be so much more meaningful and long lasting.

I will say to other CKD patients, that both types of dialysis were very inconvenient and took a huge toll on my body physically and emotionally. Back in 1993, I did not know anything about living donor kidney transplants. In fact, I knew little about the difference between dialysis and deceased-donor transplants, let alone the difference between deceased donor transplants and living donor transplants, which can give the recipient nearly double the years of function. I now see how important it is for patients to be more proactive, that is if you and I want to live our best life possible.

I was blessed with a second chance of life through my second kidney transplant, gifted to me from the heart and body of my living kidney donor and the love of my life and wife, Kim, on March 5th, 2009.

I am so grateful. I am in awe every time I think about it because without Kim's generosity my life's outcome would be very bleak. I would be subjected to hemodialysis 3 times a week and sit for 5 hours at a time. I would arrive home weak, tired and lifeless. I'm convinced I would have died connected to that machine.

I'm extremely and eternally grateful for this 2ʳᵈ chance at life, a life that is dialysis in-dependent. This story is even more special when I appreciate how Kim and I met and how long we have known one another. We met when we were in high school back in 1969. Even back then Kim knew we were supposed to be together. She would tell me often that she came into my life for a reason. We decided to get married and start a family in 1989. Her insight to the enormity of the role she now plays in my life today is quite magical, to say the least.

This experience has caused me to pause and never take this gift of life for granted. I hope to inspire other potential recipients through my story, so they can live their best life too by choosing living donor transplant over dialysis.

I also hope my story will encourage patients, like the ones I met through the years I was on dialysis, so they know there are other options--better options. I want them to stop settling for less, like most of us do when we don't know any better.

And most of all, I wish to publicly acknowledge "the love of my life" Kim, for saving MY life and enriching our union. Because of her, my life is abundantly blessed. This incredible life-changing experience has transformed my life and my expression of gratitude at the deepest level of my core.

-Ryan P.

Transplant Recipient Story #3

I guess my story starts back in 2002. I was in California attending a small community college in the Sierra Nevada's. I went in to the doctor to get a prescription for attention deficit disorder medication, which was prescribed to me. They decided to do a full work up and physical since I had not had one in a long time. The blood test showed my creatinine level was high.

The doctor proceeded to tell me that my kidney functioning (GFR) was at 40 percent and that eventually I would have to get a transplant or dialysis. I thought "Wow!" I just came into to get some medicine and I received this very heavy and discouraging news. Here I thought I was a healthy twenty one year old, who plays soccer, skateboards, hikes, stays physically fit, and who was so healthy, I didn't even need to see a doctor, or so I thought.

This was big and daunting news. I decided to shut myself off to it for a several years. I would tell myself, "I feel fine. This can't be happening to me. I'm young it won't catch up to me until I'm much older."

Through test and ultra sounds and a review of my medical history, it was discovered that the cause of my kidney disease occurred at birth. I had Ureter Reflux when I was born and had surgery to fix it when I was about three weeks old. This caused urine to spill back into the kidneys causing scarring, which as time went on, caused my kidneys to work harder, which led to their gradual decline in function.

I left California a short time after and enrolled into college at Oklahoma State University, where I'm originally from. The move was, in part, a path to get back on my parents medical insurance, so I could see nephrologists regularly. In Oklahoma, I was referred to a local nephrologist who monitored my function and educated me on the five stages of kidney disease. I was shocked to learn I was already at stage three.

That's about all the information I received, no information about transplant, no information about dialysis, no information about where this was going to go. So, once *again, I chose to believe I was "good to go" for another long while, since no one told me otherwise.*

If I would have known then what I know now, I would have been a lot more proactive in finding out what my options were, but nothing had been explained in any detail to me. Information is power and I didn't have the information to empower myself with it at the time.

At the age of twenty five, I was kicked off my parents insurance. I had a hard time trying to find insurance with my pre-existing condition. Then, I discovered that I could get insurance through the Oklahoma State University as a student, if I paid a higher premium. That lasted about a year until I graduated college. During that year I started having high blood pressure, so I was given a medication that seemed to level it out for a while.

While uninsured, I avoided nephrologist visits because I couldn't afford it. I also believed I was still doing fairly well and that everything would be fine.

By the next time I went to see a doctor, my function had deceased to twenty-two percent and my blood pressure was a problem again. I had dropped to one of the lowest levels of stage four in less than a year and a half. I was just seven points away from dialysis!

It wasn't until my the doctor called with the results, that it finally hit me. "I really am sick and I'm about to go on dialysis!" This was super scary news. Needless to say, I started seeing nephrologists on a regular basis again, yet this time I became proactive, I received and read all the information that I was given on kidney disease, and I grilled my doctors for more information. I went online and did my own research, and found great resources. The National Kidney Foundation was a huge resource of information and support.

I started learning what it would be like to go on dialysis. And what life would be like to receive a kidney transplant instead. By this time I was married and I was able to get on my wife's insurance plan, no questions asked.

That summer, my wife and I moved to Phoenix, AZ, for an internship that my wife had accepted. So I started seeing a local nephrologist in Phoenix, who was much more actively involved than any of my previous doctors I had seen. He strongly urged me to get on the transplant list at Mayo Clinic, because they had one of the biggest and most successful transplant facilities in the United States. By this time I was down to around seventeen percent function and had been listed on UNOS's national waitlist. The current average wait time for a kidney was 3-5 years. It was then that I learned of living kidney donation.

I think one of the things I struggled with most was how to approach people about living kidney donation. Basically, I was told, just ask. I did talk about it to my family and close friends, but most people didn't know I was even in need. So I resigned myself to the fact that I would have to wait it out for a deceased donor.

When my wife finished her term in Phoenix, we moved back to Texas. Then, I received a phone call that would completely change my life. It was so surreal and just three months after getting on the list. I was told by Mayo Clinic that I would be receiving a kidney from a living donor who altruistically wanted to donate her kidney to someone in need. We ended up being a perfect match, so I was moved to the top of the list. I flew back to Phoenix and went into surgery on the 27th of December.

Now, I have to mention this here, because before surgery I had read a lot about how some people feel instantly *better. This usually occurs with patients who have been on dialysis. Since I hadn't, I figured it probably wouldn't apply to me. To my surprise and delight, I felt 50 times better! My head was clear, I wasn't tired at all like I usually am, and my energy was springing forth even after a major surgery. If I could have ran around the hospital jumping for joy, I would have. I felt that different.*

It really started to impact me just how amazing it was for me to be given a second chance at life. I truly feel blessed. It's hard to imagine a random person whom I've never met, gave life to me. I was released in two days from the hospital, mainly because of my young age and because I was healing fast and the organ was working amazingly well.

Honestly the biggest impact I felt was pure generosity of my donor. Now, I want to help people. I want to help others understand the process better and get through all the misleading information so they know what their options are.

Recently, I joined the National Kidney Foundation's PEER Mentor group to provide phone support to people with chronic kidney disease. I hope to help them avoid the issues that I had to go through and to give them some hope. I also wanted to share my story here with you, so you could see that things aren't at all as daunting as they appear. Transplant Medicine has come a long way in the last thirty years.

I am three weeks post-transplant as I write this story. I am full of energy and loving life. I am not going to waste this gift that has been given to me. If I could leave you with one piece of advice it would be: "You are your strongest advocate. Take advantage of it. Speak out and be heard."

-Granger B.

Forms, Charts & Scripts

Lab Chart Snapshot

MY LAB CHART

TEST	DATE	DATE	DATE	DATE
CREATININE				
GFR				
BUN				
ALBU SERUM				
HGB				
HCT				
RBC				
WBC				
PLATELET COUNT				
NA				
K				
CL				
CA				
PHOS				
MAG				
ANION GAP				
GLUCOSE				
AST/ALT				
CHOLESTEROL				

Blood Pressure Log

BLOOD PRESSURE LOG

TIME/DATE	SYSTOLIC	DIASTOLIC	PULSE

Body Awareness Log

BODY AWARENESS LOG

DATE/ TIME OF DAY	DESCRIBE SENSATION	CAUSE SUSPECTED	LEVEL OF DISCOMFORT
			PAIN SCALE **1-10** (10 BEING WORST) 1-2-3-4-5-6-7-8-9-10
			PAIN SCALE **1-10** (10 BEING WORST) 1-2-3-4-5-6-7-8-9-10
			PAIN SCALE **1-10** (10 BEING WORST) 1-2-3-4-5-6-7-8-9-10
			PAIN SCALE **1-10** (10 BEING WORST) 1-2-3-4-5-6-7-8-9-10
			PAIN SCALE **1-10** (10 BEING WORST) 1-2-3-4-5-6-7-8-9-10
			PAIN SCALE **1-10** (10 BEING WORST) 1-2-3-4-5-6-7-8-9-10
			PAIN SCALE **1-10** (10 BEING WORST) 1-2-3-4-5-6-7-8-9-10

OUTREACH TRACKER

CONTACT NAME	EMAIL ADDRESS	DATE SENT	FOLLOW UP DATE	STATUS

Your Buddy's Story Script

"My friend/wife/colleague has chronic kidney disease which is rapidly squelching his/her remaining kidney function. He/she needs a kidney transplant from a living kidney donor, or he'll/she'll be forced onto dialysis for an undetermined amount of time.

Currently, there are over 100,000 people waiting in line ahead of [insert name] on the national kidney transplant list. Sadly, the average wait for a kidney from a deceased donor is several years. [Insert name] can't wait that long without risking their life.

Living donors help those in need by giving them a healthy kidney when they need it most. The only wait when a living donor offers, is the time needed for donor testing, transplant committee approval—and God willing, the surgery date.

While I was hoping that I could be his/her donor, I was told I would not qualify due to my health history. This is why I'm sharing his/her story in hopes to find a potential living kidney donor who would qualify. I'm sure there someone out there who would be a viable donor and a good match. I also believe there are those who seek extraordinary opportunities in human kindness.

Please help me spread the word about [insert name]'s needs so we can increase our circle of influence.

With Sincere Gratitude,

E-Blast Your Story

Dear friends of [insert name]

Thank you for taking the time to read this very important email about our mutual friend [insert name]. I am writing you to update you on the serious medical challenge he/she is facing right now to see if you can help.

[insert name] is in (urgent) need of a kidney transplant. I was hoping to be his/her donor, but due to various medical reasons I am unable to participate. [insert name] family has also been denied this opportunity, so this is why I am extending our reach in communication.

Usually when someone is dealing with a critical health problem, all we can do is support them—and believe me, that's needed here too. Yet this time, there is an opportunity to save a life. Since I have been told that I cannot be the one, I'm hoping to create BUZZ so the message expands our circle of influence by making this need become more universally known.

Currently, there are over 100,000 people on a list waiting for a kidney ahead of [insert name] and their average wait for a deceased organ donor's kidney is nearly five years. This wait causes more than a dozen deaths a day.

[insert name] can't wait that long without serious health risks. If [insert name] doesn't get a kidney transplant soon, he/she will be forced to be tethered to a dialysis machine, just to stay alive.

Living donors can end the wait. There have been over 125,000 living kidney donor surgeries performed, so this is not new. We just need to get the word out, because there might be a potential donor out there who isn't aware of this opportunity.

Please feel free to contact me for more information. Thank you again for taking the time to read this very important email.

*Please forward this email to others, to further expand our efforts.

Written Intention Statement

Intention Statement

I, Risa Simon, received a living kidney donation offer from a remarkably vibrant and healthy living kidney donor during the month of April 2010. My donor has been fully tested and approved by my transplant center as an ideal donor and match for me. My surgery was scheduled in an efficient and timely manner, which allowed me to bypass the need for dialysis.

My body instantly recognized my new kidney as a "part of me" by instinctively accepting it and protecting it as one of its own from the moment it was connected.

Both surgeries were a huge success, followed by smooth and speedy recoveries. The only impact my donor feels post-procedure (other than the short period of expected post-surgical discomfort) is endless pride and joy for their remarkable life-saving act of human kindness.

I celebrate this gift-of-life daily with profound respect and gratitude. My new kidney continues to provide me excellent renal function—and a quality of life most can only dream of. I am now living that dream.

And so it is.

Risa Simon

Donor Script –Announcement To Family

Ice Breaker:

"Does your driver's license show you're an organ donor? Hey, look here. So does mine! That means we're both organ donors! Something we can both be very proud of, eh?

I recently registered my wishes with the State online as well, on the www.organdonor.gov page, after I discovered that's the more official way to make our wishes known. It's easy and I can help you with that if you'd like.

Have you ever given much thought to living organ donation? I'm referring to donating a kidney to someone in need today while you're still alive? Have you ever thought about that? Did you happen to catch that story in the news the other day? So inspiring, don't you agree?"

Intro:

"Those stories really got me thinking. I can't imagine a more selfless or courageous act of human kindness than that. Can you?

I'm really intrigued with the thought of doing something like that now, while I'm in the prime of my life and healthy enough to do so. It just sounds like such a meaningful goal to achieve. It would be a shame to hold back everything until after I die, when I can do something now. I want to live the rest of my life knowing how I contributed to something bigger than myself. (pause)

Support Your Position:

I've done a lot of research and learned that the surgery is laparoscopic, meaning very small incisions and quicker recovery. Most donors are out of the hospital the next day and back at work in three weeks.

The surgery appears to be no more dangerous than any surgical procedure done under general anesthesia, and all medical expenses related to testing and the surgery are covered by the transplant recipient's insurance."

I also discovered that there is no scientific evidence in the 50 years of living kidney donation history that there are any ill effects to living with one kidney. And over the last 23 years of tracking the statistics, there have been over 110,000 living donor transplants performed.

Evidently the remaining kidney increases in size and filtering power to match the power of two kidneys. So, in essence, the donor has one turbo-charged kidney instead of two normal ones. It's as if we were intended to have a spare for this exact purpose! (pause)

I also discovered that kidney disease typically affects both kidneys, so the thought of needing a spare for ourselves, really doesn't come into play much, unless someone has developed kidney cancer or experienced bilateral trauma. I know I don't have a crystal ball, but I don't think those are high risk factors for me due to our family history or my lifestyle. (pause)

Another great discovery is that if the donor ever needs a kidney down the line, they basically go to the front of the waitlist line, because they already donated. Currently, there are over 90,000 people waiting for a kidney and the average wait is nearly five years. No one can wait that long when they need a kidney today. A living kidney donor is the only way those in need can end their wait."(pause)

Express Your Desire/Intention

"I recently met a person who is in urgent need of a kidney.

Usually when someone is critically ill, all we can offer of ourselves is our love and support. But here, I can do so much more. I could save a life—or, at the very least, give someone a life worth living. (pause)

I've been told that a kidney transplant from a living donor can function twice the number of years than a kidney from a deceased donor.

I realize you might need some time to process this conversation, but I'd just wanted you to know that I really want to do this and it would mean the world to me to have your support.

Your thoughts and feelings matter to me. Actually, they matter a lot. I'd like us to have an open exchange about your feelings without the fear of upsetting one another. (pause)

I'm going to leave some resources and related materials so you can do some investigation of your own if you'd like. Perhaps we can talk again in a day or so. Would you be open to that?"

Donor Announcement Letter

Dear Family and Friends,

I have something important I'd like to share with you and I know that it might sound a bit wild. It has to do with my desire to help someone who is in need of a kidney transplant. For some time now, I've felt an inner jab to do something bigger than myself, but I wasn't sure what that might be. When I learned about the possibility of saving a life by becoming a living kidney donor, I was almost immediately captured by this purposeful call.

I'm writing you because I wanted you to know that I'm looking into this. I still need to see if I would be healthy enough to do so. For now, I simply wanted to share this information with you since you've played a key role in my life. It is out of my love and respect for you that I'm seeking your blessing.

In case you're wondering, I've done my homework and researched the process thoroughly. And though you may not understand my motives at this time, please know that I have not been influenced or coerced into doing this. This decision was triggered by me, shortly after I discovered there was someone in need.

Your opinion and future blessing would mean a lot to me. Please share your thoughts so I may address them by providing additional information and resources.

And while I realize that we may never see eye to eye on this, I do hope if I'm approved as a match and if I'm healthy enough to proceed, that you'll be able to cheer me on without too much concern.

I also hope (within time) that you'll see my desire to donate one of my kidneys as a once-in-a-lifetime opportunity to serve mankind. No doubt, it will be the greatest and most meaningful achievement of my life.

RESOURCES & LINKS

Patient Support, Mentoring & Coaching

1. The Pro*active* Path
    Private & Group Coaching, Workshops, Seminars & Webinars
    4757 E. Greenway Rd, Ste 107b-25
    Phoenix, AZ 85032
    480 575 9353
    Email: Risa@TheProactivePath.com
    web: www.TheProactivePath.com

2. National Kidney Foundation Peers Program
    Patient Education Support Network & Peers Mentoring Program
    30 East 33rd Street
    New York, NY 10016
    800 622 9010
    Email: Kelli.Collins@kidney.org
    Web: www.kidney.org

3. Renal Support Network
    Patients Helping Patients: Education, Support & HOPEline
    Glendale, CA 91207
    www.rsnhope.org (800) 579-1970

For Statistics, Data & Resource Links

1. U.S. Department of Health & Human Services (HRSA)
    Organ Procurement and Transplantation Network (OPTN)
    Access & research transplant data
    http://optn.transplant.hrsa.gov/data/

2. Scientific Registry Of Transplant Recipients (SRTR)
    Find A Kidney Transplant Center & Calculate Your Wait Time
    Administered by: the Chronic Disease Research Group
    A Minneapolis Medical Research Foundation
    914 S. 8th Street, Minneapolis, MN 55404
    www.SRTR.org (Phone: 877-970-SRTR)

3. Centers for Medicare and Medicaid Services (CMS)
   U.S. Department of Health and Human Services
   Use this link for information on: Medicare and Medicaid
   Information & Benefits
   www.medicare.gov/navigation/medicare-basics/medicare-benefits/medicare-benefits-overview.aspx

Educational Resources

1. National Kidney Foundation
   Patient Education, Mentoring & Support
   30 East 33rd Street
   New York, NY 10016
   800 622 9010
   www.kidney.org

2. American Association of Kidney Patients
   The Voice of All Kidney Patients For Education & Support
   2701 North Rocky Point Drive, Suite 150
   Tampa, Florida, 33607
   800 749-2257
   www.aakp.org

3. TransplantFirst Academy
   Proactive Patient Engagement for Renal Groups
   & Transplant Centers
   4757 E. Greenway Rd, Ste 107b-25
   Phoenix, AZ 85032
   480 575 9353
   Risa@transplantfirst.org
   www.transplantfirst.org

4. The Proactive Path
   Patient Coaching, Seminars, Webinars & Books
   4757 E. Greenway Rd, Ste 107b-25
   Phoenix, AZ 85032
   480 575 9353
   web: www.ThePROactivePath.com

5. National Kidney Center (NKC)
    Online Kidney Community for Information, Options & Hope
    20081 Whistling Straits Place
    Ashburn, VA 20147
    703 662-1253
    www.nationalkidneycenter.org

6. The American Society of Transplantation
    Clinically Focused Information About Transplantation
    15000 Commerce Parkway, Suite C, Mt. Laurel, NJ, 08054
    Use this link to learn more about how AST is advancing the
    field of transplantation
    www.a-s-t.org

7. KidneyLink
    News Reports & Valuable Information on Kidney Transplantation
    Managed by the PKD Foundation
    8330 Ward Parkway, Suite 510
    Kansas City, MO 64114-2000
    800-PKD-CURE
    www.kidneylink.org

8. KidneyKinships
    Outreach Website
    4757 E. Greenway Rd #107b
    Phoenix, AZ 85032
    www.kidneykinships.org

Educational Resources – Living Kidney Donors

1. TransplantFirst Academy's LKD Tribute Campaign
    Outdoor Living Donor Awareness Campaign - Educates &
    Inspires Communities to Consider Living Kidney Donation
    4757 E. Greenway Rd, Ste 107b-25
    Phoenix, AZ 85032
    480 575 9353
    www.1Kidney.org

2. American Living Donor Network (aka - ALDF)
A Project of the Center for Ethical Solutions
Helping Living Donors & Recipients
40357 Featherbed Lane
Lovettsville VA 20180.
info @ helplivingdonorssavelives.org

3. National Kidney Foundation – Big Ask, Big Give
Providing information for living donors
30 East 33rd Street
New York, NY 10016
800 622 9010
www.livingdonors.org

4. National Living Donor Assistance Center (Financial)
Provided by HRSA to reduce financial disincentives to living organ donors
2461 S Clark Street, Suite 640
Arlington, VA 22202
888.870.5002
www.livingdonorassistance.org

5. United Network for Organ Sharing (UNOS)
Uniting & Supporting Patient Communities
"Living Donation: Information You Need To Know"
www.unos.org/docs/Living_Donation.pdf

6. California Pacific Medical Center
New! Educational video on living kidney donors
2340 Clay Street, San Francisco, CA 94115
415-600-1700
http://www.cpmc.org/advanced/kidney/LivingDonation/

7. The Department of Health and Human Services
Division of Transplantation
200 Independence Avenue, S.W.
Washington, D.C. 20201
877-696-6775
www.organdonor.gov

8. Living Kidney Donor Network
   Workshops, Webinars & Informational Resources
   Living Kidney Donation
   312 473-3772
   www.lkdn.org

9. University of Michigan, Transplant Center
   1500 E. Medical Center Drive
   Ann Arbor, MI 48109
   Information on donation and transplantation
   www.TransWeb.org

10. Emory Kidney Transplant Program's
    1365 Clifton Road, NE, BLDG B, 6th Floor
    Atlanta, GE 30322
    404-727-3250
    Download Living Kidney Donor Pamphlet:
    www.emoryhealthcare.org/transplant-center/pdf/living-donor-brochure-kidney.pdf

Paired-Donation Programs

1. Alliance For Paired Donation
   3661 Briarfield Boulevard, Suite 105
   Maumee, Ohio 43537
   877. APD.4ALL
   www.paireddonation.org

2. UNOS-United Network For Organ Sharing/Paired Donation
   700 N. 4th Street
   Richmond, VA 23219
   (804) 782-4800
   https://www.unos.org/donation/kidney-paired-donation/

3. The National Kidney Registry
   P.O Box 460
   Babylon, NY 11702
   800 401-8919
   www.kidneyregistry.org

Suggested Reading – Information/Inspiration

1. Kidney Disease: A Guide for Living
   By Walter A Hunt & Dr. Ronald Perrone
   The Johns Hopkins University Press
   http://www.amazon.com/Kidney-Disease-Living-Walter-Hunt/dp/080189963X

2. Preemptive Renal Transplantation: Why Not?
   Informative article on Preemptive Renal Transplants
   Manage, Kevin C.; Weir, Matthew R.
   http://onlinelibrary.wiley.com/doi/10.1046/j.1600-6143.2003.00232.X/full

3. United Network for Organ Sharing (UNOS)
   "Living Donation: Information You Need To Know"
   www.unos.org/docs/Living_Donation.pdf

4. When Altruism Isn't Enough:
   The Case For Compensating Kidney Donors,
   By Dr. Sally Satel, AEI Press
   Use this link to access Dr. Sally Satel publications
   http://www.sallysatelmd.com

5. Brilliant Eats - Delicious Recipes To Be *KidneyWise*™
   www.pkdcure.org/hardgoods/brilliant-eats-cookbook.html

6. The Reluctant Donor
   A Live Donor's Journey
   By Suzanne F. Ruff
   www.thereluctantdonor.com

7. The Untethered Soul
   A Journey Beyond Self
   By Michael A Singer
   A New Harbinger Publication
   wwww.newharbinger.com

INDEX

R

S

T

About the Author

The highlight of **Risa Simon's** life was the day an unexpected, unrelated, living kidney donor offered to give her a kidney – and tests revealed a sister-like match. That day didn't come easy, and it might never have come at all, if she wasn't willing to become a proactive contender, competing for her best life possible.

Risa knows all too well what it's like to be a kidney patient trapped in a hopeless sinkhole, worming its way to dialysis. As she watched her numbers decline, her emotions escalated. Like many patients, she felt paralyzed by her loss of control.

Then, by a stroke of luck, she attended a kidney patient conference and experienced the most profound awakening of her life. This personal awakening empowered her to jump off the kidney disease conveyer belt and start proactively fighting for her best life possible. As told in this book, her transformative journey turned into a powerful platform of proactive strategies. Her intention was to create a plan that could help all those in need, not just herself.

Today, Risa is living her best life ever. Her gratitude and unwavering resolve to help her book fans, clients and mentees compelled her to step away from a successful consulting and speaking career. Her vision was to fully immerse herself into the renal community. That's exactly what she did and she's never looked back.

Her ultimate dream was to create a proactive platform to inspire patient empowerment through speaking engagements, coaching and mentoring. She also dreamed of starting a non-profit 501c3 organization that partnered with renal groups and transplant centers who wanted to advance educational curriculums and inspire their patients to seek a transplant before dialysis.

Her dreams came to life after establishing the TransplantFirst Academy www.TransplantFirst.org and The Proactive Path www.TheProactivePath.com. On any given day, you'll find Risa advocating to empower kidney patients to seek better outcomes. Her unwavering commitment to help others is enthusiastically portrayed in her passionate obsession for this calling.

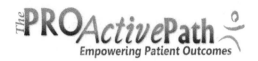

For More Information on Speaking Engagements, Private Patient Coaching & Workshops:

The Proactive Path
A Division of Simon Says Seminars, inc.

www.TheProactivePath.com
info@theproactivepath.com

TRANSPLANTFIRST
EMPOWERED PATIENT ACADEMY

TransplantFirst Academy
A 501c3 non-profit organization
www.TransplantFirst.org
risa@transplantfirst.org

<u>How To Order More Copies of This Book:</u>
This book is available in Paperback & Kindle in Amazon's Online Book Store; or by visiting: www.ShiftYourFate.com

Made in the USA
Las Vegas, NV
07 May 2022

48545442R10157